HERBAL DISCOVERIES

Nona-Michael Ankhesenamun Jackson

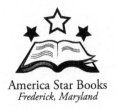

America Star Books
Frederick, Maryland

First printing

America Star Books has allowed this work to remain exactly as the author intended, verbatim, without editorial input.

This publication contains the opinions and ideas of its author. Author intends to offer information of a general nature. Neither the author nor the publisher are engaged in rendering medical, health or any other kind of personal professional services to the reader. The reader should consult his or her own physician before relying on any information set forth in or implied from this publication. Any reliance on the information herein is at the reader's own discretion.

The author and publisher specifically disclaim all responsibility for any liability, loss, or right, personal or otherwise, which is incurred as a consequence, directly or indirectly, of the use and application of any contents of this book. They further make no representations or warranties with respect to the accuracy or completeness of the contents of this work and specifically disclaim all warranties including without limitation any implied warranty of fitness for a particular purpose. Any recommendations are made without any guarantee on the part of the author or the publisher.

Softcover 9781681228075
PUBLISHED BY AMERICA STAR BOOKS, LLLP
www.americastarbooks.pub
Frederick, Maryland

CONTENTS

CHAPTER ONE

THE HERBAL COMBINATION FOR BREAST CANCER: FENUGREEK

Breast Cancer is believed to be more of inherited than a sudden disease. Breast cancer, like every other terminal illness, however comes from not taking the appropriate herbs to prevent toxins and free radicals that affect daily lives.

Breast Cancer is believed to be more of inherited than a sudden disease. Breast cancer, like every other terminal illness, however comes from not taking the appropriate herbs to prevent toxins and free radicals that affect daily lives.

Breast Cancer is such, that it begins to accumulate toxins and like every other organ, results into an illness.

The breasts have to be taken care of in a much more hydrated way. Bathing daily and doing basic hygiene is good but having regular mud bath and exfoliation are the vital ways to beat cancer. To beat cancer, the need to take daily herbs are essential.

Fenugreek serves many purposes. It works like the herb called Sage Leaf, by relieving the stomach of internal gas and indigestion. Fenugreek also contains Lecithin that breaks down bad fat, making it useful for cholesterol and blood sugar regulation.

Fenugreek also contains fibre, making it a cleanser for the intestines. This means that the Fenugreek shares some working qualities with Acai Daily Cleanse pill.

Fenugreek is one of the main ingredients in preventing and curing breast cancer. Fenugreek also nourishes the breasts, giving it back its breast tissues as older age begin.

There may be more than one herbal combination for breast cancer cure as time goes on. With new herbs, come new mixes and with new mixes, come better discoveries.

a. The herbal combination for Breast Cancer and Fenugreek include: Hydrolysed Collagen which drains out toxins and excess fluids through the lymphatic drainage system.

b. Herbs for breast cancer combination also include St John's Wort, Lemon Balm, Royal Jelly, Sage leaf, Water Balance, Cranberry, Aloe Vera Colon Cleanse and Ashwagandha.

c. St John's Wort is an excellent herb for reducing breast tumors and on a very high and recommended dose, it destroys the tumor or cysts in the breasts. Taking the herbal combination with Evening Primrose Oil, is also essential.

d. Regular yoga exercise is excellent. Using the gym is brilliant but must be minimal especially for a person with terminal illness. The body needs strength and replenishing to re-start the immune system and heavy gym usage may cause tragic consequences.

CHAPTER TWO

THE HERBAL COMBINATION FOR THE TEETH: SPIRULINA AND TOOTH CELLS

The teeth has various problems at any age. Whether as a teenager or as a growing adult or at older age. During youth, and when the teeth is stronger is the time to begin the herbal intake of Calcium and Magnesium.

Herbs and minerals that ensure healthy growth and maintenance of the teeth keep the teeth stronger as youth gives in, to older age.

Getting older is a good thing when the body is kept youthful and healthy. The teeth is working all the time and it begins to weaken in time. There are many herbal combination for the teeth. In fact, the teeth has the largest herbal combination in the world because of its functions.

Spirulina is one of the main ingredients that the teeth need all the time. Taking this mineral often should ensure stronger bones and suppleness between the gum and the tooth.

The Spirulina contain herbs and minerals that contain tooth cells and repairs broken tooth whilst strengthening it. The avoidance of tooth removal can be achieved when time is taken to care for the teeth with natural herbs, organic mouth wash and organic toothpastes.

The herbal combination for the teeth is more complicated than any part of the organ of the body. The tooth might be in pain today, because its tissues are wearing out. The tooth might be in pain, because it needs Calcium and Magnesium to keep it stronger.

A terminal illness complicates the strength of the teeth and therefore taking a high dose of the relevant herbs and minerals will eventually strengthen the teeth. This could take a year or more, depending on how high the immune system is boosted, regularly.

Putting mercury in the tooth makes the tooth weaker. The dental instruments may weaken the tooth and even cause injury later on. Then, there are other facts to consider: what happens when the next tooth begins to ache? Should every tooth be removed, every time there is a pain?

Dental instruments may weaken the jawbone in time. Mercury may begin to stray into the digestive tract and into the stomach causing internal problems. Although Chromium Picolinate and some herbs remove metals and toxins, inside the body, it is best not to have mercury there. Mercury of that nature, is foreign to the tooth and unnatural.

The Spirulina remineralizes the tooth and restores its tooth cells. A normal tooth in need of tooth cells may take some forty eight hours or more to complete the remineralization process, depending on the dose and number of times, the Spirulina is taken.

Hydrolysed Collagen repairs the teeth, as well as the bones in the body. Water Balance is useful for the teeth because it flushes out excess fluids. But draining fluids out of the body, also mean replenishing it, too.

A combination of Hydrolysed Collagen, Spirulina, Glucosamine Sulphate, Water Balance, N-Acetyl-Cystein, Amino1500, Vitamin C, Complete B Complex, Ashwagandha, Aloe Vera Colon Cleanse, Black Cohosh, Oil of Peppermint, St John's Wort and L-tyrosine help to maintain the teeth's strength.

CHAPTER THREE

THE HERBAL COMBINATION FOR SKIN CANCER, CANCER AND ALL TERMINAL ILLNESSES: ASHWAGANDHA

Ashwagandha is the herb that works like natural botox. It is positively assumed as THE TREE OF LIFE. Perhaps it was its seed that made it through, after the flood assumption. Wherever Ashwagandha herb has come from, it is the watch word for eternity.

Ashwagandha works for all terminal illnesses, flu, colds, bites, acne, stress, jet lag, long train travels, and ageing.

A skin cancer can be cured by taking Ashwagandha as a main ingredient. The Ashwagandha can also prevent the amputation of the legs. This herbal combination include: COQ10 Enzyme, Quercetin with Vitamin C, Evening Primrose Oil, Lemon Balm, Hydrolysed Collagen, St John's Wort, Garlic Oil, Complete B Complex, Brewer's Yeast, Garlic Oil, L-Glutamine, L-Tyrosine and Ashwagandha.

A terminal illness does not necessarily mean that the skin has no more hope. Instead, the Ashwagandha makes healing possible, thus, keeping the chemical injections and chemical botox injections away. However, a natural Organic Botox injection containing non-synthetic medicine such as Ashwagandha may speed up the good skin results.

When a person is terminally ill, the skin may be difficult to respond to healing. However there is a reason behind this. It is generally assumed that until you have cancer, you are not carrying cancer cells. In fact, any type of terminal illness makes you a carrier of cancer cells.

In the case of diabetes, you already have cancer cells spreading into the body system. The cancer cells in diabetes are not as rapid as the cancer diagnosis themselves. Actually, the cancer cells in diabetes are more subtle and would have infected the entire body organ system in the same speed as cancer.

Unknown to the diabetic, the cancer cells are in the body system; but slowly destroys the inside of a person. It is why diabetes is filled with all sort of complications the moment it infiltrates the body system. It is why there are still complications long after a person goes into remission.

Removing any part of the organ may not prevent cancer returning but flushing out cancer cells and its toxins keep the body organs working as if in youth.

Oiling the skin shold be done with organic creams and lotions that are completely free from parabens and synthetics.

CHAPTER FOUR

ASHWAGANDHA AND STRESS

Ashwagandha is the herb that ultimately treats stress. Stress levels can be caused by a number of factors. It could be from typing, housekeeping and gardening, driving, fishing, carrying heavy groceries and general chores.

Stress being the first signal to a cardiac arrest or liver disease, begins slowly but steadily. If treatment is not taken within, it may increase the blood sugar and blood pressure, which results in diabetes. This is where Ashwagandha becomes very useful, but this herb might as well be, the STRESS-FREE drug.

Without stress, there probably will be no illness.

Ashwagandha is not just for skin cancer, but also for hair growth, voluminous hair growth and natural hair color.

Ashwagandha is a main herb for a singer's voice. It improves the singer's voice, the vocal chords, enhances the speech and moistens the mucous membrane. This is why there is less sneezing, catarrh and colds when taking Ashwagandha.

The herb Ashwagandha is best taken in the evenings and when not operating a machinery. It is also best taken with Black Cohosh because it consumes a lot of Estrogen and testosterone.

Ashwagandha is useful for the skin because it heals the stress that causes the ageing and the wrinkling of this skin.

Relaxing the muscle with Ashwagandha, Valerian root and ginger root are also helpful while observing daily siesta.

CHAPTER FIVE

ASHWAGANDHA AND BLACK COHOSH

Although Ashwagandha is used for arthritis, it should be combined with Black Cohosh, Evening Primrose Oil and Glucosamine Sulphate because it saps fluids and Estrogen. The herb also stabilizes the blood pressure and the blood sugar.

Ashwagandha may restore barrenness especially after a terminal illness such as cancer. However, it cannot be used alone because it saps estrogen. Therefore, Ashwagandha should be taken with Black Cohosh, Agnus Castus, Vitamin C and sometimes, Resveratrol.

Ashwagandha aids a good night's sleep. The herb should not be taken on its own. Although it is a sedative, it should be taken with Vitamin B, Ginger root and amino tablets.

Like Ashwagandha, Sports Nutrition herbs sap endocrine hormones such as testosterone, estrogen and collagen, therefore, the way to restoring the herbs would be by taking Black Cohosh which contains estrogen, garlic oil, essential oils and hydrolysed collagen amongst herbs and minerals that restore the endocrine hormones.

Yet, the sports nutrition herbs, restore these very endocrine hormones that they protect.

CHAPTER SIX

ASHWAGANDHA OR L-5-HYDROXYTRYPTOPHAN

Ashwagandha or L-5-Hydroxytryptophan are essential ingredients when treating a person for any illness including, a heart attack. However, they cannot be taken alone:

a. Ashwagandha with Black Cohosh OR L-5-Hydroxytryptophan with Ginger root.

b. Ashwagandha with Aloe Vera Colon Cleanse and ginger root

Ashwagandha with Uva Ursi. The Uva Ursi can be taken for up to seven days or as directed.

In some cases, directed dosage of L-Glutamine with Ashwagandha and ginger root may help resuscitate a cardiac arrest patient. This is because glutamine expands the blood vessels to increase blood circulation to the heart although it has been personally known to do this best on high dosage.

e. A patient waking up from a surgery may have some discretional L-Tyrosine injected in the glucose or its alternative because it clears the throat of fat blockages thus, increasing respiration.

f. Sometimes, L-Hydroxytryptophan is preferred instead of Ashwagandha. They are both sedatives and work in similar ways although Ashwagandha is more traditional.

Ashwagandha may aid slimming but should be combined with Black Cohosh, Lemon Balm, Sports nutrition and St John's Wort. Water Balance and Brewers Yeast are the main ingredients for water weight loss.

Skin Cancer like most cancer start to heal almost immediately, after taking Ashwagandha. This takes a year to three years after which, it should be taken often. Stress is never far away and so, Ashwagandha should be kept close. Make it your best friend because Ashwagandha itself is like an Island.

CHAPTER SEVEN

ASHWAGANDHA: NUMBER ONE HERB

Withania Somnifera, also known as Ashwagandha, is the number one herb, for every illness.

Ashwagandha calms the mind, body and soul. It relieves from mental disorders, nervous disorder, panic disorders or bipolar disease and epilepsy. Best taken with herbs, minerals and vitamins such as vitamin C.

Ashwagandha is also a blood cleanser and fights virus completely. Best taken with garlic oil and aloe vera colon cleanse pill.

Ashwagandha cleanses the blood best, with Aloe Vera Colon cleanse. The Aloe Vera Colon cleanse is a blood thinner, so to speak, and may cause dizziness so that it should be taken with a sedative such as L-hydroxytryptophan, Valerian root or Ashwagandha.

Although Ashwagandha may prevent a mental disorder and breakdown, it should be taken with sage leaf, ginger root, cranberry, cod liver oil, vitamin c and evening primrose oil. It also helps a person with skin irritation, allergy such as water allergy and complications caused by diabetes.

CHAPTER EIGHT

ASHWAGANDHA AND INJECTIONS

Ashwagandha herb is good for skin healing after injections, injections from blood samples, surgical needles from drips, insulin injections and regular injections. It begins by healing the nerves and the weakened veins. The herb should be taken with Complete B Complex and Brewer's Yeast. A previously weakened vein, can however take up to a year or two to complete healing especially after a terminal illness and depending on the strength of the immune system.

To make healing faster, take sports nutrition herbs such as L-Glutathione, L-Glutamine that may help break down the fat to allow an increase in blood circulation. The weakened veins are supplied with nutrition that speed up the strength thus, brightening the skin again and boosting its rejuvenation. You can add herbal tan tablets to make the skin glow incredibly and why not enjoy herbal creams, lotions and body butter to make healing more effective.

Stress weakens the bones so, when working, it is best to take Calcium and Magnesium; Glucosamine Sulphate and Spirulina regularly and possibly daily or as recommended.

By using the gymnasium, the muscles may weaken in time and therefore need sports nutrition regularly. Minimize the using of the gym and where possible, enjoy yoga and aerobics. Go to a ballet dancing class and enjoy more of flexible movements rather than tedious gym equipments that weaken the bones and muscle in time.

When taking herbs, vitamins and herbs, it is best not to take synthetic drugs and chemicals because the herbs can work in their own right. The herbs work best for terminally ill persons, at high doses. The immune system of some patients break down completely to the point that such a person has to take up to two hundred pills a day. Until the immune system recovers, it is always best to maintain high doses.

If there is a suspected overdose, immediate intake of Aloe Vera Colon Cleanse and Water Balance should be taken.

CHAPTER NINE

ASHWAGANDHA AND ADRENAL GLANDS

Ashwagandha increases the brain cell production and when taken with Resveratrol, it stabilizes the Adrenal glands. There is the neurotransmitter in the brain that causes depression, stress and fatigue when its level is low. However, the herbs calm and control all types of fatigue and syndrome that may occur.

The Adrenal gland which is located on top of the kidneys play a major active role in the entire body system. It is where stress begin and even ends. A little sign of stress, is a little big problem.

The Adrenal Gland is connected to the Superoxide found in the brain. The superoxide is responsible for the connective tissues between the brain, the brain cells and the Adrenal gland.

When there is an infection in the body system, it is the Adrenal gland that responds immediately and the response could be as tragic as the ending. It could begin as itching, with boils, acne and sudden weakness. Ashwagandha maintains the body's immune system, however, the herbs should be taken with other recommended herbs and vitamins such as Vitamin C because it may stop the breathing, just as easily as it can improve the breathing and mucous membranes.

The immune system is heavily dependent on the digestive tract system. The main herbs for the digestive tract are: Ashwagandha, L-Tyrosine, Brewers Yeast, Milk Thistle, Ginger Root, Oil of Peppermint, Sage Leaf and N-Acetyl-Cysteine.

The adrenal gland is also connected to the skin and gives brightness and shine to the skin when taking in a combination of ashwagandha, garlic oil, tan tablets, pycnogenol, resveratrol, Brewer's yeast, hydrolysed collagen, cod liver oil and L-glutamine.

The human body is severely deficient of most herbs, vitamins and minerals and it is why the body is prone to toxins and terminal illnesses. It is also why the body's need for herbs is raised so high in dose, when it comes to herbal intake.

Oxidative stress in humans are far higher than thought. This is because, from the moment we wake, to the moment we start the first blink, pull the bed covers or duvet aside and then get out of bed, we are already working. We are already stressing and by lunch time, we are stressed, yet stress may not be felt until one day, when it is too late.

Just getting out of bed, making tea or hot chocolate, making breakfast, to reading a newspaper, are slow but steady stress moves. When herbs are not taken daily, these stress become heavier and then we are wondering why. We wonder because we have not lifted a heavy weight bag or item but we have walked about, we have cooked meals and we have tidied the house.

Those who type daily on the computer, are especially at risk of sudden collapse. People who sit behind a desk and type for hours, especially long hours, may find the symptoms almost immediately. The legs may be in pain but you may think nothing of it, until you feel that you cannot do anything about it. Yet, Chromium Picolinate, Brewer's yeast, ashwagandha and a complete sports nutrition alleviate these problems.

This is why many people have leg problems. Why many people are in wheelchairs, why many people use crutches. It is because they do not take vitamin c daily. Hydrolysed collagen, sports nutrition such as L-Arginine help open the blood vessels so that proper circulation can be accomplished.

Those who take amino 1000 in a combination of amino acids that make the protein, will understand that the dose have to be high enough to attain real goals.

High amino herbal intake may cause the blood volume and platelets to be too high. When taking amino herbs, take with water tablets, Brewers yeast and essential oils.

Calcium with Magnesium is vital because magnesium ensures that the body system is receiving this strength and should be combined with Spirulina that is yet many times stronger than Calcium. This would mean that Calcium is still a critical mineral even on its own and yet it cannot function thoroughly without magnesium by its side as per combination.

CHAPTER TEN

ASHWAGANDHA AND SERUM GLOBULIN

The Adrenal glands are responsible for the normality of the Serum Globulin; on whether the Serum Globulin is normal, slightly high or very high. The Ashwagandha and the Garlic Oil work with the white cells in the body to attack infection. However, Ashwagandha can take years to complete its attack on infections that have full blown cancer and terminal illness such as Diabetes.

A herbal intake that includes sport nutrition herbs, help remove fat toxins from the body. Tan tablets are highly lipid soluble and are especially good for the vision. However, it is recomended that tan tablets be taken with garlic oil and ashwagandha because it may induce apoptosis.

Ashwagandha may be useful for the thyroid glands although, it is best to take this herb with Evening Primrose Oil and L-Tyrosine and N-Acetyl-Cysteine when treating the throat and the lungs.

The serum globulin levels may not return to normal basically because of high cholesterols and fat toxins that must be flushed out of the system. This is the reason why a person with a healthy thyroid gland or organ, but who may be obese, may suddenly go into a cardiac arrest or have congestive heart failure. The body is under a false security when it is not been cared for all the time.

A little indigestion is a warning, a morning sickness may be a mini alert system, regurgitating while eating or drinking may be a sign. Yet, a test may be carried out and the body is fine. The reason is not that you have been thrown a voodoo spell.

The reason might actually be a gradual deterioration of a body organ especially the thyroid glands.

The endocrine system of the body is exceptionally sensitive and may not give any immediate warning before a sudden collapse, but would have been given you a symptom, that most likely would have been bypassed because of its seeming irrelevance, which could be as insignificant as a cough or a hiccup or a mild pain in the chest that came as quickly as it had hit.

Yet, the sports nutrition herbs are there to protect the body that especially is obese. The sports nutrition keep the thyroid glands healthy and protect the digestive system from heart burns. The proper health is a daily care regime and would be treated daily as if having a daily meal at least. The sports nutrition work best when combined with ashwagandha and necessary herbs, vitamins and minerals.

CHAPTER ELEVEN

ASHWAGANDHA AND CARTILAGE TISSUES

Ashwagandha is also useful for the joints but as useful as it is, to the joints, it is also capable of causing osteoarthritis, when taken on a long term. To take the Ashwagandha for long, it is best taken with Glucosamine Sulphate, Vitamin C, Cod Liver Oil and Calcium with Magnesium to heal the joints, and maintain the fluids and cartilage tissues.

Ashwagandha saps fluids in the joints and yet, it also heals the joints. It is why it should be taken with a Sulphate, Calcium and Spirulina or a bone strengthening herb.

CHAPTER TWELVE

ASHWAGANDHA AND COLLAGEN TISSUES

Ashwagandha may sap collagen tissues from the teeth. It may cause occlusion when it saps tooth cells. The teeth is made use of daily because of eating and chewing and therefore it needs replenishing daily. When taking Ashwagandha herb, take with Water Balance, Hydrolysed Collagen, Spirulina, Sulphate and Calcium should also be taken.

Water Balance saps fluids especially in a diabetic, so shoud be taken with L-Glutathione or N-Acetyl-Cysteine.

Collagen is very important in the body and for the bones and body tissues. It is also crucial for the lymphatic drainage system where the breasts are taken care of, as excess fluids are flushed out of the system.

The breasts must be cared for daily, by taking Evening Primrose oil, Fenugreek and other necessary herbs, minerals and vitamins that prevent excess fluids from forming hard lumps made of toxins.

CHAPTER THIRTEEN

ASHWAGANDHA AND DAILY HERBAL INTAKE

These are a lot of herbs to take in at any one day, but every individual has to understand how their body should work. Perhaps, alternating herbs weekly might be best:

a. Monday: Ashwagandha, Ginger and Hydrolysed Collagen

b. Tuesday: Ashwagandha, Ginger and Spirulina

c. Wednesday: Ashwagandha, Ginger and Calcium with Magnesium and Vitamin D

D. Thursday: Ashwagandha, Ginger and Glucosamine Sulphate or Sulphate

e. Friday: Ashwagandha, Ginger and Silica

f. Saturday: Ashwagandha, Ginger, Turmeric and Hydrolysed Collagen

g. Sunday: Ashwagandha, Ginger, St John's Wort and Calcium, Magnesium and Vitamin D.

FOLLOWING WEEK:

a. Monday: Ashwagandha, Ginger root and L-Glutamine

b. Tuesday: Ashwagandha, Ginger root and L-Arginine

Wednesday: Ashwagandha, Ginger root and Amino100 tablets

Thursday: Ashwagandha, Ginger root and L-Glutathione

e. Friday: Ashwagandha, Ginger root and tan tablets

Bone strengthening herbs, vitamins and minerals are quite strong and hard, as they should be. Although they should be taken daily, care shoud be taken as to saturation and when adding other herbal medicines.

CHAPTER FOURTEEN

ASHWAGANDHA AND SAGE LEAF

Taken Ashwagandha daily and Sage Leaf may also mean taking them at different times of the day, especially because both do cause some drowsiness.

Ashwagandha is important because it maintains the blood levels in the body. This prevent dizziness and fainting.

Sage leaf cures the cough, sore throat and gum disease. It also is a natural mouth freshener. It generally reduces body sweat and odor.

CHAPTER FIFTEEN

ASHWAGANDHA AND IRON

Sometimes, the body especially the fingers, get a shock when metals are touched especially on cold days. It might be because the body temperature is so low or that there is insufficiency in Iron content in the body. Ashwagandha may prevent the lack of blood flow that may cause the body to react to metals and certain objects. Ashwagandha contains Iron.

The mineral called Potassium also helps to stabilize the blood but should be taken on low dose because of its very high potency.

Instead of taking Potassium directly, it can be take as L-Tyrosine which contains Potassium.

Organic moisturisers help alleviate shocks and shingles that may have been caused by a lack of potassium in the body to stabilize the imune system.

CHAPTER SIXTEEN

ASHWAGANDHA AND SUPER GUARANA

Ashwagandha is also useful for shingles but best combined with Super Guarana.

Ashwagandha is so vast in work, that in time, it cleanses off scars, birth marks, spots, acne and tattoos. It is a very strong herb and should be taken with other herbs, minerals and vitamins and as recommended.

Ashwagandha is also used for softening the skin when taken on a high dose. The skin is smooth and bright, and slowly but steadily cleanses the varicose veins. This should be taken with the equally powerful St John's Wort and ginger root.

Ashwagandha may cure headaches and migraine but it is best taken with St John's Wort and Essential Oils.

CHAPTER SEVENTEEN
ASHWAGANDHA AND VARICOSE VEINS

Varicose Veins can be cleansed from the body softly, gently and with time. However, a person with terminal illness will realise the lethal potency of varicose veins, perhaps, even too late. Varicose Veins is one of the major complications in an illness. It easily turns the varicose veins to a large wound filled with cancer cells and toxins.

As a result of varicose veins, there could be an amputation or death of blood circulation in the area. To prevent this major disaster, it is best to take Ashwagandha regularly, oiling the body with organic creams. Care should be taken by regularly oiling the skin with organic creams and Vaseline. Cocoa butter and Shea butter are useful and beneficial so as to prevent the spread of the wound.

Particular care should be taken to the side of the waists and hips; the anal area should be cleaned with a wet pice of towel and then dried with a clean one, then oiled, to prevent hemorrhoids.

The breasts and under the breasts should be generously oiled daily, and the inner thighs should be cleaned with a warm towel, dried and nourished with oil.

Adding Sage Leaf to the Ashwagandha regime is also essential. The Sage Leaf herb help the skin to relax and stay calm, especially when under the blankets and duvet at nights. By perspiring in a stable condition, the skin stays healthy while excess perspiration lead to skin sores, wounds, itching and more severe problems.

CHAPTER EIGHTEEN

ASHWAGANDHA AND CARDIAC ARREST

When a person has a heart attack or heart disease, Ashwagandha may be given in low doses with Aloe Vera Colon Cleanse Pill and Water Balance pill. This method of healing a heart patient is natural and may help a person with Cardiac arrest to recover, without side effects to the brain and organs.

Fibroids should be controlled by taking Acai Daily Cleanse pill, Water Balance, Lemon Balm, St John's Wort, Cranberry, Ashwagandha and Aloe Vera Colon Cleanse. Fibroids of the good type should be maintained so that they can capture the toxins and excess fluids thus flushing them out of the body and preventing a cardiac arrest.

Discretion should be noted when given ashwagandha because it is a sedative that yet waken the brain's cells. Dose will vary per person and healing time will take time and effort.

CHAPTER NINETEEN
ASHWAGANDHA AND SORE THROAT

When having treatment for an illness, it is always best to take the full package to avoid infection in other areas of the body. A mere sore throat can easily cause sorrow to the entire body system.

Sore throat has a package because it carries the infection through the digestive system to the intestines, urinary tract and anal area. The herbs therefore will prevent side effects and toxins. Herbs for sore throat include: L-Lysine, Cranberry, St John's Wort, Lemon Balm, Sage Leaf, Ashwagandha, Oil of Peppermint, L-Glutamine, Aloe Vera Colon Cleanse and Full Digestive Enzyme.

The digestive system has to be cared for daily because of the regular swallowing when eating and drinking. The cartilage need to be serviced in other words. The tissues in the digestive tract should be maintained with bone active herbs to give them the strength to continue.

Oil of Pepperint aids better digestion especially when taking daily tablets.

CHAPTER TWENTY
SAGE LEAF AND ODOR

Sage leaf is useful for the digestive system, stops bad breathe, minimizes farting and bad odor, prevents mouth odor, urine smell, armpit odor, menstrual odor, excretion odor and general skin and body odor. It regulates sweat and calms at nights.

Basically, St John's Wort works in similar ways as Ashwagandha thus preventing infection although these herbs have to be taken in high doses to work best.

CHAPTER TWENTY-ONE
ASHWAGANDHA AND OBESITY

Obesity can be prevented by taking a combination of sports nutrition and herbs. An obese person can trim and slim slowly but steadily by taking high dose of St John's Wort, Lemon Balm, Ashwagandha, Royal Jelly, Hydrolysed Collagen, Sage Leaf, L-Lysine, Aloe Vera Colon Cleanse pill and Oil of Peppermint.

Aloe Vera Colon Cleanse pill may lower the strength of the brain and heart circulation and should be taken with Ashwagandha, ginger OR L-5-Hydroxytrptophan with ginger root.

For colds, catarrhs and sneezing that may come from changes in the body because of slimming, it is best to take Turmeric, St John's Wort, Water Balance, Vitamin C, Complete B complex and Ashwagandha.

CHAPTER TWENTY-TWO
ASHWAGANDHA AND DIABETES

Ashwagandha herb fills the holes in the uneven skin, under the skin, and the uneven hair scalps.

Diabetes is a slow killer. It keeps the sufferer, in a state of suffering. But diabetes can be cured. The complications from diabetes is far worse than the lethal diabetes itself. The moment the blood sugar rises, it spills from the pancreas to the kidneys and into the urinary tract system.

It takes a little spill of blood sugar and the body is gone unless control is found. A little spill of blood sugar detected, and put in control immediately may still be as lethal because complications begin almost instantly.

Diabetes carries cancer cells that slowly destroy the body while cancer itself is faster and rapid. Detoxifying the pancreas every three months or as required is important. Take Uva Ursi for seven days and every three months to keep the pancreas in function and prevent pancreatic cancer. It also protects the kidneys and maintains the heart and circulation.

The pancreas can be re-started by taking a combination of Brewer's Yeast, Zinc, Beta-Carotene/tan tablets, ashwagandha and Complete B Complex.

Diabetes without painful complications make the sufferer think that they are safe. This is far worse on the longer run because diabetes is a slower form of cancer which slowly but actively generates cancer cells that may cause full blown cancer when not controlled.

Diabetes is a complication of all illnesses. An irritable bowel syndrome to a diarrhea problem to a cold or flu is a complication of diabetes and may need various herbs to bring it to control.

Diabetes and Diarrhea is a case of stomach upset that never seem to expire. Constant diarrhea reduces the strength of the muscle and fibres and may cause stomach cancer if not treated.

The Sage leaf helps to tighten the stomach muscles. The loose stool may refuse to change to bulkier stools. The loose stool may be in green or other color. The stomach becomes a disruptive and noisy place when the herbal combination is not taken as it should. Cranberry also tightens the stomach walls and should be taken with sports nutrition such as L-Glutamine.

Eating normally is best whether a person has diabetes or is in normal health. However, when a person is not losing the weight especially on the scale monitor, there would be a need to increase the sports nutrition and do some yoga.

Sports nutrition such as L-Glutathione, L-Glutamine may be increased in many ways:

2000mg capsules every hour for four hours and every day for a month to six months, depending on how obese a person is.

Most sports nutrition are 500mg per capsule which would mean that up to four capsules per hour should be taken.

CHAPTER TWENTY-THREE
ASHWAGANDHA AND UVA URSI

Uva Ursi is also useful with Ashwagandha as it speeds up the healing process of wounds, varicose veins and cellulite incurred during a terminal illness. The wounds destroy the nerves, causing shingles, pain, swollen foot and severe irritation.

It is possible that multiple sclerosis develops and this could result in bone collapse. Taking Ashwagandha, Calcium, Magnesium, Spirulina, Resveratrol, St John's Wort, sports nutrition pills or powder, Vitamin C and Hydrolysed Collagen may improve cognitive powers.

Uva Ursi is one of the many leading herbs that attack infection and cancer cell. Uva Ursi basically starts the healing of the wound. This beginning is a serious step and the right herbs should be taken in addition, so as to energize the wounded area to further responsive treatment.

CHAPTER TWENTY-FOUR
ASHWAGANDHA AND THE CORTISOL LEVELS

The Cortisol levels should be checked regularly because this is the steroid hormone that is released from the adrenal glands to reduce stress and regulate the pituitary gland in the brain.

The Ashwagandha aids the steroid hormone levels to stabilize so that there is sufficiency working in the body. Ashwagandha being an adaptogen energizes the body on a daily basis. It is a stress fighter and unique.

Sometimes, the anal area may itch and cause irritation. Ashwagandha softens and smoothes the area from hemorrhoids. The Ashwagandha should be taken with Aloe Vera Colon Cleanse pill.

While Ashwagandha is a most powerful herb in the world, it only helps with major recovery until the rest of the illness is given better care. However, you never need to stop taking Ashwagandha because of free radicals.

Ashwagandha will help a terminally ill patient recover so as to be in remission but that is only the beginning. Shedding the excess weight is another major factor to consider. Ashwagandha is there to prevent more toxins in the body and to eliminate toxins in the fat. Shedding bad fat helps the Ashwagandha to work better while health and strength improves.

CHAPTER TWENTY-FIVE
ASHWAGANDHA AND SEX

Ashwagandha is good for the urinary tract and should be taken with Cranberry and St John's Wort. It keeps the area fresh, healthy especially after sexual intercourse.

During a terminal illness, a person might want to exercise. A diabetic may want to exercise to shed weight and bad fat, however the taking of things slowly and calmly is essential.

A diabetic may do simple exercises that will not complicate the illness such as yoga and walking. Too much exercise may be consequential. However, there is hope in Ashwagandha, Sports nutrition pills and powder and Complete B complex and Brewer's Yeast.

CHAPTER TWENTY-SIX
ASHWAGANDHA AND DIABETIC CURE

The most powerful herbs to cure Diabetes of any type are: Ashwagandha, Complete B complex, Brewer's Yeast and St John's Wort. Sports nutrition should be taken with Ashwagandha and ginger root or with L-5-Hydroxytryptophan.

St John's Wort destroys all the toxins and viruses in the body system when taken regularly and at high dose. Lemon Balm destroys bad bacteria that may be found in the intestines and colon. It helps the bile to work properly so that it breaks down foods for small intestine digestion.

The strongest amino acids for the small intestine are the L-Glutathione and the L-Glutamine. L-Glutathione is excellent for the small intestines however, it may also lighten the skin. For proper and better swallowing via the digestive system, L-Tyrosine should be added in the combination.

To achieve greater value and quality when slimming down, amino acids or sports nutrition are best taken with garlic oil of 1000mg x 6 every hour for at least six hours in a day. This is also an incredible way of enjoying a better life in remission.

To maintain the hair or for balding problems especially during a terminal illness, a combination of essential oils, amino acids, herbs, minerals and vitamins are most effective in the right dose and with the right combination.

Like all medicines, always check with your Herbal Practitioner before taking any medicine.

Diabetes is linked to the thyroid glands and the endocrine system. When the thyroid glands stop working properly so that the metabolism slowly collapses, it is when illnesses such as diabetes occur. Basically, it is not the eating that causes the diabetes nor is it necessarily the fat that causes the diabetes, but the collapse of the endocrine system especially the thyroid glands.

You probably can eat as you like as long as the metabolism is working properly and bad fat is flushed out of the body system.

A person with a large adams apple may find that it reduces in size as they take amino acids, protein shakes because sports nutrition slim and trim body fat while increasing the muscle mass.

CHAPTER TWENTY-SEVEN
ASHWAGANDHA AND BLOOD PLATELETS

Ashwagandha is a herb that increases the blood platelets when it is very low. A number of reasons could cause low blood platelets such as insufficient white blood cells, mosqito bites, fever and leukemia. Ashwagandha should be taken with Fenugreek and Complete B Complex. Aloe Vera Colon cleanses the blood of toxins and blood clot, Garlic Oil fights infection and increases the white blood cells. It should also be taken with Quercetin and Vitamin C because Quercetin cures spider bites, snake bites and poison.

St John's Wort may also be added to increase the blood platelets as it restores the muscle calmness so as to aid the increase and it is also good and protective from bites and poison.

To increase the blood platelets, Spirulina is also good because it has Vitamin K and contains fifty times more of Calcium.

Brussels Sprouts is good for the blood and also good for the Pancreas. Spinach is fresh and acts as a healthy detox.

Ashwagandha helps to de-stress tooth that may be swollen or loose. The tooth and the gum must be appropriately located otherwise, it becomes loose.

Stress may cause gum to be swollen. The water balance pill is very useful for Pyorrhoea and may help strengthen the teeth.

Herbs such as Siberian Ginseng, Chromium Picolinate and Zinc should be taken separately from Ashwagandha, which also acts as a blood tonic.

Ashwagandha, amino acids, Cranberry and Acai Daily cleanse are good herbs for bulk excretion and for removal of toxins from the walls and arteries.

It is believed that fat and obesity cause diabetes and cancer. It is possible that bad fat cause high cholesterol levels thus causing a terminal illness. Fat in itself contributes to the heart disease and excess toxins, because bad fat is not breaking down to be flushed out of the system.

CHAPTER TWENTY-EIGHT
ASHWAGANDHA AND THE KIDNEYS

The Kidneys serve a lot of purposes in the body. They cleanse the blood and help remove excess wastes and fluids in the body. Urine is produced in the kidneys and the kidneys have to be working properly to allow wastes out of the body system.

Ashwagandha rectifies the damage that may have been caused by little bile production. The bile aids the breakdown of fat and foods through the intestines and that is why the excretion is in brown color. The depreciation in bile may lead to celiac disease and green excretion and this can damage the wall linings of the small intestines.

For a person with a terminal illness, there is a faster chance of the kidneys filling up with wastes to be flushed out of the system. This should be maintained by taking water balance and cranberry tablets regularly at a dose that may be higher than one for a normal healthy person.

Amino acids remove bad fat within months when taking on reasonably high doses. Taking amino acids or any medicine must be supervised. Amino acids are unpredictable as to speed when it comes to the metabolism and this is why it is best to take all medicines with Ashwagandha and ginger root or L-5-Hydroxytryptophan with ginger root.

The amino acids are the most powerful for the endocrine body system and work through every birthday of any life span.

CHAPTER TWENTY-NINE

ASHWAGANDHA AND MILK THISTLE

Taking Milk Thistle with Ashwagandha may rectify the damage and restore proper excretion. For better and healthier excretion it is also best taken with Acai daily cleanse pill which contains Psyllium husks and green tea.

The bile has to be working properly to aid the digestion of fats, calcium and Iron otherwise it leads to osteoporosis because of a lack of absorption.

Milk Thistle cannot be taken on its own, at least, it is recommended to be taken with Ashwagandha, Calcium, Magnesium and Vitamin D because of its high potency that may cause dizziness.

Milk Thistle increases the hair growth of the eyelashes and eyebrows.

CHAPTER THIRTY

ASHWAGANDHA AND GLUTEN

A person who has Celiac disease may take Ashwagandha, Milk Thistle, St John's Wort and Lemon Balm to rectify the issue but eat gluten and dairy with caution. Celiac disease may be cured by taking from the herbal package that include sports nutrition, protein shakes, with meals regularly.

A Celiac disease sufferer may want to add Agnus Castus to the herbal combination because it may sometimes cause irregular menstrual period.

Sometimes, the stomach is troubled and there might not be an immediate way of knowing what is going on, in there. Therefore, the herbal intake of Uva Ursi may be useful for the period that the pain exists. If pain continues after many hours, it is likely that the bile is not functioning properly and may need Ashwagandha, Milk Thistle, Sage Leaf, Acai daily cleanse pill, Oil of peppermint, Calcium with Magnesium, L-Glutamine and Glucosamine Sulphate to rectify the problem.

CHAPTER THIRTY-ONE
ASHWAGANDHA AND ACAI DAILY CLEANSE

Acai daily cleanse pill cleanses the fibre walls from toxins and helps with bulky stool.

The bile is made up of bile salts, bilirubin, electrolyte and phospolipids. The bilirubin must be kept clean, with its test level kept normal. This is because an over-filled bilirubin might lead to the recycling of dead and old cells that should be excreted as wastes. The Turmeric is the powerful herb included in this exceptional combination of body purification.

Sometimes it may not be the bile with the problem, it may be the kidneys. It may be that the kidney stones are sticking in the walls of the urinary tract and causing great pain. The kidney stones, which is made up of minerals and salts stick together rather than get flushed out of the body. It becomes a problem as the salts and minerals begin to form pebbles that may cause vaginal itching and appendicitis on the long run.

Salts and minerals must not stick to the wall linings in the urinary tract. These should be excreted out and flushed out as wastes because they are toxins that have been flushed out of the kidneys already.

To correct the issue, Ashwagandha, Cranberry, St John's Wort and Complete B complex with Brewer's Yeast should be taken. The Chromium Picolinate is another powerful ingredient that flushes out stubborn metals in the body system. There is Chromium in Brewer's Yeast, however.

CHAPTER THIRTY-TWO

ASHWAGANDHA AND VERY HIGH HERBAL DOSES

Ashwagandha is particularly useful for a person with cancer. In very high doses of Ashwagandha, cancer can be controlled and cured. It may involve high doses of herbal mixes that could be up to two hundred pills taken from a week to three weeks. After three weeks or even less, the dosage is reduced or spread out some more.

High herbal doses are needed to overpower cancer and bad fat. Aloe Vera Colon Cleanse is so strong in its cleansing work and soothing of the anal after heavy stool, so much so, it cannot be taken on its own.

It is advisable not to discontinue the Ashwagandha unless otherwise stated. Doses may be reduced for the herb and in fact, any other herb, long after remission occurs to avoid free radicals and radioactivity effects.

CHAPTER THIRTY-THREE

ASHWAGANDHA AND MUD

With a terminal illness, it is best to use body mud to wash the body frequently, organic exfoliation and hydration of the skin are all contributory factors that aid the body's immune system to return to normal. Body mud, hair mud however, reduce the strength of the immune system, so that Ashwagandha or L-5-Hydroxytryptophan with ginger should be taken before and after treatments.

As a matter of fact, cancer treatment with herbal medicine work best when combined with the use of mud products.

CHAPTER THIRTY-FOUR
ASHWAGANDHA AND DAILY SKETCH SAMPLE

A rough herbal plan for a cancer patient may look like this:

Day 1: Ashwagandha x4 every thirty minutes for six to eight hours, taken with ginger x4 every thirty minutes for eight hours.

Day 2: Ashwagandha x4 with ginger x4 every thirty minutes, alternating with Uva Ursi x4 with Complete B complex x4 every thirty minutes for eight hours or more.

Do note that individual's may reach saturation earlier than expected and must reduce the dosage. Perhaps, spacing the time of next intake to every hour. Your Herbal Practitioner would know how.

Day 3: Ashwagandha x4, Sage Leaf x4, ginger x4 every thirty minutes alternating every thirty minutes with Uva Ursi x4, Complete B complex x4, Vitamin C of 1000mg x2 for eight to ten hours.

Day 4: Ashwagandha x4, Glucosamine Sulphate x4, ginger x4 every thirty minutes with Complete B complex x4, Acai Daily cleanse x4, Uva Ursi x4 for eight hours.

Day 5: Ashwagandha x4, Calcium with Magnesium with Vitamin D x4, ginger x4 alternating every thirty minutes with Complete B complex x4, Sage Leaf x4, Uva Ursi x4 for up to eight hours.

If saturation occurs, overdose or regurgitation is felt, Aloe Vera Colon Cleanse and Water Balance should be taken starting with x1 each. Although, it is always expected that the intake of any medicine should be supervised and directed.

Day 6: Ashwagandha x4, Spirulina x4, ginger x4 alternating every thirty minutes with Complete B complex x4, Uva Ursi x4, Acai daily colon cleanse x4 for up to eight hours a day.

Day 7: Ashwagandha x4, Hydrolysed Collagen x4, ginger x4 alternating with Brewer's yeast x4, Uva Ursi x4 and Uva Ursi should be taken for up to seven days only unless otherwise stated; Sage Leaf x4 for up to eight hours a day.

The regime can alternate every week however,Ashwagandha and Complete B complex must be maintained every week whether the dose is low or high.

CHAPTER THIRTY-FIVE
ASHWAGANDHA AND THYROID GLANDS

Thyroid glands are located in the neck. This is where the metabolism becomes sensitive and need care and caution. Sometimes, the metabolism is moving faster than it should perhaps, there is a life changing situation or a new weight loss programme. Whatever is causing the thyroid glands to make a sudden move to speed up, a process known as Grave's disease, can be rectified with herbs.

Ashwagandha, Evening Primrose Oil, Cod Liver oil, Brewer's yeast, Aloe Vera Colon cleanse pill, Zinc and Sea Kelp are some of the main herbs that improve the thyroid glands. Iodine containing herbs are all useful.

The thyroid glands produce hormones called thyroxine and triiodothyronine that control the growth and metabolism of the body. The glands must be working properly to avoid overactivity or low activity of the glands.

When carrying a bag or heavier item, always take Evening Primrose oil and Cod liver oil to balance the sudden circulation and fat breakdown that may occur.

The amount of fat breaking down in the body and in the neck must balance with the amount of bad fat and toxins being flushed out of the body. Taking the herbal combination and having some form of simple yoga exercises may help restore balance. Having Burdock tea, green tea, Dandelion tea may also help with the proper circulation in the body.

CHAPTER THIRTY-SIX
ASHWAGANDHA AND SEA KELP

When taking Aloe Vera Colon cleanse or Sea kelp, always take with Ashwagandha and ginger root OR L-5-Hydroxytryptophan and ginger root. Basically, Sea kelp may cause sudden speed of the metabolism which may cause dizziness.

CHAPTER THIRTY-SEVEN
COD LIVER OIL AND PROTEIN

Cod liver oil is a vitamin that can be taken with Ashwagandha to firm the stomach and produce protein. It may firm the skin and the elasticity of it. Cod liver oil may also firm the intestinal area to aid bulkier stools rather than loose ones.

Cod liver oil strengthens the shoulders and the chest especially when losing much fat in the breasts and its surrounding area.

CHAPTER THIRTY-EIGHT

ASHWAGANDHA, COD LIVER OIL AND RICKETS

Cod liver oil contains vitamin A and D. This helps the vision and increases the sharpness and brightness of the eyes as well as regulate the neurotransmitter in the brain.

The Cod liver oil contains vitamin D which is useful in firming the bones and preventing rickets. Without the vitamin D, the possibility of the stomach collapse may occur, because the muscles in the stomach begin to weaken and may reduce the strength of the intestines in producing bulky stools. It may also reduce the strength of the bile in breaking fat and calcium.

The vitamin D in Cod liver oil also helps the stomach to be more at peace with itself so that it can work properly.

The Cod liver oil may aid relief for diarrhea and inflammatory bowel syndrome. This should be taken with Ashwagandha, Aloe vera colon cleanse which prevents ulcerative colitis, Sage leaf keeps the proteins together and make them supple; Oil of Peppermint soothes the gastrointestinal tract and St John's Wort destroys infection.

Ashwagandha also strengthens the bones, the teeth and when in need of strengthening the bones, it is Ashwagandha, you want and need. For a very soft bone leading to osteoporosis, taking Ashwagandha x4 every one to two hours for some six hours for four days strengthen the bones. An Herbal Practitioner would be consulted before taking any medicine.

CHAPTER THIRTY-NINE

ASHWAGANDHA AND POTASSIUM

Sometimes when it is cold and the skin touches metal, there is a sense of shock. However, taking Spirulina which contains Potassium helps to reduce such an effect especially on cold days.

Avoid taking Potassium on its own because of its high potency and speed to saturate. L-Tyrosine is also an amino acid that contain Potassium and is protective of the body's electrolyte system.

CHAPTER FORTY

ASHWAGANDHA AND HAWTHORN

Where possible, avoid taking Hawthorn on its own but if it has to be taken, it should be done with supervision. Hawthorn regulates and strengthens the heart, so it is a useful herb but must be taken with ginger root and vitamin C. After taking Hawthorn, take Ashwagandha within that hour or as directed. L-Glutamine is a sports nutrition that strengthen the heart and the chest.

However, taking herbal medicines in single forms, may not be as effective as taking them in relevant combinations or in high doses. For example there might be little or no results achieved when taking Vitamin C x1. But taking Vitamin C of 1000mg x3 tablets or x4 tablets is bound to heal a swollen feet when taking every hour for six hours or more a day.

CHAPTER FORTY-ONE

ASHWAGANDHA AND PALM LINES

The palm lines tend to have so-called creative designs on them during a DNA collapse. There are strange drawings and lines on the palms, strange chain like designs that seemingly look like thin bracelets around the wrists.

The strange designs caused by a DNA collapse may cause severe irritation and may signify a terminal illness and a form of cancer. This can be brought under control when Ashwagandha, garlic oil and Turmeric are taken.

Turmeric with Tan tablets are also useful for the skin and smooth out such 'drawings' on the palm lines thus, restoring the DNA cells to normal in the herbal combination.

Sudden movements and longer movements may cause distress to the body causing sudden breakdown of fat. While it is significant that there is a fat breakdown, it is also essential to monitor such, so as to avoid a situation whereby more fat is breaking down while the body begins to wobble because of a lack of balance and steadiness.

This should be rectified immediately with face and body exfoliation, Ashwagandha and ginger root, sports nutrition and protein drinks to regulate the body fat and fluids.

The palms must be fresh, smooth and clear. The only birth lines on the palms are probably three or four lines. In time, study may find that lines probably shouldn't be on the palms at all or they should be fainter.

CHAPTER FORTY-TWO
NONA COMPLETE HEALTH REGIME

THE NONA COMPLETE HEALTH REGIME: The combination of the regime is as follows:

Yoga as recommended, optional gymnasium exercise <twice a week> is not necessarily recommended for a person who is already in strenuous work or who is ill. This is why the yoga is best as exercise although there are other forms of exercise such as skipping, dancing, karate, horse and pony riding, golf, brisk walking and shopping.

Daily herb pills and tablet intake of Ashwagandha and ginger root or 5-hydroxytryptophan and ginger root are essential because of sudden extra movements, and new herbal intake that may take the time to absorb and adapt to the body system.

Herbs are taken without synthetic drugs, hydrating the skin is vital for healthy pores, exfoliating <such as with Apricot face and body scrub containing Elderflower>, exfoliating with salt scrubbing salts such as with salts from the Israel's Dead Sea and sugar scrub.

Mud mask for the face and body mud detox eliminate toxins, the mixing of Emollient cream with organic toning creams may alleviate eczema and othe skin problems.

The mixing of vaseline and organic creams help smooth out the skin from varicose veins and skin distress.

Organic foot and heel scrub and creams protect the feet and the heels. Soaking the feet daily in salts or oils are so relaxing and blessed.

Organic and herbal toothpastes and mouthwash keep the mouth healthy as they work with natural herbal medicine. Non-Steroidal Emollient cream, help metabolize the liver so that it continues to work as normal.

Unhealthy creams soak up the liver and reduce its proper functioning. This may cause toxins to swell causing an illness.

Emollient creams may also be massaged into the body, with tea tree lotion, Aloe Vera gel, UVB, organic Cocoa butter creams, Natural Shea butter,Aromatherapy oils <such as sweet almond oil, Miaroma oil>, optional Sun moisturizing lotions may be rubbed into the body with discretion, because they are said to sap vitamin D. The daily intake of Vitamin D3 and Cod liver oil might just be better but if in doubt, why not take tan tablets which are quite good for the vision.

Eating of foods and drinking in moderation is an obvious recommendation. Eating a piece of cake that is less than 20g of saturated fat and has less than 90g of sugar, a day, does not necessarily cause an illness. It is the lack of health regime and herbal intake that cause the illness.

A can of pepsi or coke may not cause diabetes or an illness when combined with healthy herbs and regime. Flushing out wastes from the kidneys may be causing the problem when not done daily. Waste may be recycled in the body when not flushed out of the liver and the kidneys.

However, the eating and drinking of low sugar products is fine. The eating of low fat and low salt foods are also fine. However, the regime may still work properly on the long run if the wastes in the body is not being cleansed out completely.

It is best to eat and drink as normal but in moderation. Diet does not necessarily restore balance and health, moderation does.

Follow your Country's fat and sugar daily guidelines for best results. Avoid too many synthetic products. Avoid synthetic hair chemicals in the hair.

Fat is said to cause Diabetes and other related illnesses. However, fat is not the main cause of these illnesses, stress is. When you are stressed, you are not caring for the adrenal glands and the endocrine system. You begin to recycle dead cells and toxins and this could result in diabetes. You are eating and drinking normally but not bothering with flushing, cleansing and detoxifying daily which can also be done by having a protein shake or a protein milk-shake.

Fat and sugar contribute and aggravate the problem in time. As the body breaks fat down, it releases toxins and spilled sugar that have been stuck in the fat. It is this fat that can cause an obese or any person, to become ill. The fat can be broken down, and as fat breaks, so must cleansing and detoxifying of the body so as to destroy virus, toxins and bad bacteria.

Bad fat may enter the bloodstream when the cholesterol is high. This is the importance of getting rid of bad fat. To maintain good fat, also take Black Cohosh and Complete B complex with Brewer's Yeast.

Have organic tea often, although organic tea may be taken with a herb and with meals. Milk Thistle tea is sometimes heavy on the legs afterwards so it is best taken with vitamin C and Evening Primrose Oil pills. This may also mean the taking of Water Balance and Spirulina which contains vitamin K.

DESSERT: Cakes and Icing-cakes with Xylitol sugar are fine. One piece of fatty cake may be the equivalent of twelve pieces of organic cakes eaten in one day. Yet, the organic cakes are rich and healthy but may be expensive.

The method of going through the entire regime regularly, whether as a healthy person or as a person in remission, is called THE NONA COMPLETE HEALTH REGIME.

CHAPTER FORTY-THREE
ASHWAGANDHA AND RESVERATROL

Ashwagandha and Resveratrol work together to rejuvenate the cells. They keep the cells youthful, healthy and fresh. They keep the blood pressure normal and prevent low blood pressure.

The Resveratrol de-stresses the kidneys, thus keeping it at work normally. The combination of the ashwagandha and the resveratrol bring the blood sugar back to normal, as if the blood sugar was never high at all.

Combining them with sports nutrition to lose all the bad fat to regulate the cholesterol is a long but steady journey. The bad fat should be coming off and if this does not show on the scale immediately it might be because there is still an ample lot of fat to be shed.

Sometimes the fat is being lost and you are visibly looking thinner but the weight is not coming off. The fact that you have noted it, is truly a good sign and beginning. You are becoming conscious of your health and you want to continue with your slimming regime until the scales are reading well.

This means that you cannot stop the weight loss regime until it is reading on the scale monitor that you are in the clear from obesity. Losing a lot of fat and no weight loss is only the beginning, because it means that you have a lot of hidden fat stored in the body, perhaps in proportionate forms like sliced cheese.

Only the scale monitor can reasonably assure you that you have lost enough weight and fat. Your cholesterol test results must be fine and normal otherwise the fat will continue to store in the body and eventually create havoc.

Slimming is about beauty, being beautiful and the scales, so do not believe anything else.

Even after losing weight and fat you still have to maintain good health and watch your test results and take your daily herbs.

A slimming plan a day, with meals, may look like this for at least four months:

Sunday: L-Glutamine 500mg x4, capsules every hour for four hours + Ashwagandha and some vitamins and minerals

Monday: L-Glutathione 500mg x4 tablets, every hour for four hours + Ashwagandha, ginger root, some herbs, vitamins and minerals every other hour

Tuesday: L-Tyrosine 500mg x4 capsules, every hour for four hours + Ashwagandha x1 + tan tablets x1 + vitamins and minerals every other hour or as needed

Wednesday: L-Arginine 500mg x4 capsules, every hour for four hours + Ashwagandha x1 + tan tablets + Essential oils + vitamins and minerals as required

Thursday: Amino 1000mg x4 tablets, every hour for four hours + Ashwagandha x1 + Resveratrol x1 + Essential Oils + vitamins as needed

Friday: Garlic Oil 1000mg x6 gel capsules, every hour for four hours + Ashwagandha x1 + Essential Oils + tan tablets x1 + vitamins and minerals as needed

Saturday: Garlic Oil 1000mg x6 gel capsules, every hour for four hours + Ashwagandha x1 + Essential Oils + Brewer's Yeast x4 every other hour and as needed.

CHAPTER FORTY-FOUR
ASHWAGANDHA AND BALDING

Ashwagandha is a basic ingredient that increases the hair volume especially in men. The testosterone levels increase as the body gets firmer. The lemon balm and the St John's Wort allow the most efficient circulation in the body to aid the growth of hair especially on bald men. Good and healthy circulation is essential for blood circulation. The bloodstream nust be clear and cleansed for proper circulation.

Lemon balm x6 capsules every hour from four to six hours with Ashwagandha will increase the chances of hair growth. St John's Wort x6 capsules every hour from four to six hours will additionally increase the power of the hair follicles. There is more guarantee in real hair growth when sports nutrition capsules and powder are added to this regime.

Rich herbal oils with dead sea mineral shampoo, serum and hair mud all contribute to the growth of the hair. Oil the hair scalp daily with the selected aromatherapy oils or herbal pomade.

CHAPTER FORTY-FIVE

ASHWAGANDHA AND ACAI DAILY CLEANSE PILL

In Chapter Thirty-One of this book, the benefits of the acai daily cleanse pill was discussed, but the acai daily has an extensive benefit and should someday, be one of the main sources of fibre value because of its nutritious content.

After smoking, the lungs may be distressed, but taking Acai Daily Cleanse pill with a reasonable dose of Ashwagandha may help. It de-stresses, cleanses and maintains the health of the lungs.

The body should be kept well even if smoking cannot be stopped. Smoking should be kept in moderation if it cannot be done without. Acai daily cleanse increases bulky stool as it saps out excess fluids from the intestinal tract.

It increases the fibre content in the body and keeps the body firmly in shape. Excess fats and fluids are removed in this way so as to give the body, better health and energy.

The Acai Daily cleanse, aids better breathing and supports a better respiratory system.

CHAPTER FORTY-SIX
ASHWAGANDHA AND ROYAL JELLY

Royal Jelly breaks fat in the liver to keep the liver healthy. When it breaks the fat, this must be flushed out by taking fibre herbs and oils so that the wastes of it does not enter the bloodstream, for it may cause heart problems.

The herbal combination should be taken with Aloe Vera Colon cleanse pill, Hydrolysed Collagen and St John's Wort. Burdock and Slippery Elm are good herbs that protect the bloodstream.

CHAPTER FORTY-SEVEN
ASHWAGANDHA AND CRANBERRY

Cranberry is good for the urinary tract. It can be taken with St John's Wort and Aloe Vera Colon Cleanse pill. Cranberry treats the urinary tract when there is no St John's Wort available.

Cranberry should be taken as frequently as possible. It flushes toxins out of the system via the urinary tract. Cranberry also removes acnes and boils from the body. It works at its best when combined with L-Lysine.

CHAPTER FORTY-EIGHT
ASHWAGANDHA AND GETTING BACK TO WORK

Ashwagandha may help in day to day life activities. At first when you take the herb, you sleep it off for a long while and then the body begins to adjust to the herb.

Getting back to work after an illness is never an easy task. But taking a herbal combination may help to find tolerance and monitor control. Ashwagandha makes this happen. Starting work for an hour to sixteen hours a week is a great motivational start in understanding the language of the body.

Either a regular sixteen hour job will be fine on the long run or just something flexible to keep both the mind and the financial mind in stability. It just depends on how the body is ready to accept this new movement. Ashwagandha may extend the life span when taken with the right herbs. With a longer life span would mean working for a livelihood.

CHAPTER FORTY-NINE
ASHWAGANDHA AND INJURY

A person taking Ashwagandha regularly may survive an accident or a crash because the blood circulation is stable and less distressed than a person who gets into a sudden crash and gets into a sudden shock or coma.

A person taken Ashwagandha may survive a coma from an accident or sudden injury, depending on how fatal the accident is. But with a herb of this nature, it is impossible to explain what a person can survive or cannot survive although it is best to always have it handy.

CHAPTER FIFTY

ASHWAGANDHA: IMPRESSION OF AN ISLAND

Ashwagandha works all on its own. If you were caught out in an Island, Ashwagandha will keep you healthy for a while. It is the Island herb that contributes to the proper healing for all terminal illnesses, colds, flu and sneezing.

It restores the hair color, it restores the skin color and the face is brighter, fresher, clearer, flawless and youthful.

Ashwagandha increases the blood flow to the hands, thus preventing Multiple Sclerosis. It also increases blood flow to the brain, thus preventing Varicose veins, epilepsy and stroke.

As good as Ashwagandha is, it is best taken, with other herbs, vitamins and minerals for proper absorption and to minimize damage to the liver and organs due to excess intake.

Ashwagandha prevents headache and it is said to be an aphrodisiac. Ashwagandha strengthens bones from fractures and increases the vision in the eyes in time. It also prevents Cataract and can be taken with the pigment-restorer capsule called the tan tablets.

Although Ashwagandha increases the fertility rate and is an equivalent to IVF treatment, it should be taken with other appropriate herbs. Ashwagandha increases sperm count and reverses impotency. Ashwagandha may reverse the menopause. It also calms painful periods.

Ashwagandha evens the teeth and the nails and prevents brittling.

Ashwagandha is especially useful for the Prostate glands, Chronic Fatigue Syndrome and memory sharpness. Ashwagandha is best taken with herbs such as Gingko Biloba and Vitamin C.

Ashwagandha may prevent and also cure Alzheimer's disease which should be taken with Complete B Complex and Brewer's Yeast.

Ashwagandha prevents and also heals stomach upset and diarrhea but should be taken with ginger root, Cranberry and Cod liver oil. It can also be used to treat appendicitis but should be taken with Aloe Vera Colon Cleanse pill.

Ashwagandha is also a greedy drug in the sense that a lot of it has to be consumed to be completely healthy.

CHAPTER FIFTY-ONE
THE RE-STUDY OF ASHWAGANDHA

Ashwagandha needs to be studied regularly. The saturated use of it may actually cause the very problem it heals. The itching and excess cortisol levels may reflect after a high dose. This should be reduced or temporarily discontinued.

Excess dose of Ashwagandha may actually cause itching again, so it should be taken with St John's Wort and Lemon Balm on a lower dose until the need for a higher dose is needed and monitored.

Excess dose of Ashwagandha or any medicine should be taken with Aloe Vera Colon Cleanse pill, Oil of Peppermint, Water Balance and Sage Leaf.

Take Acai Daily cleanse pill regularly because Ashwagandha may cause coughing. The lungs and trachea tube must be kept clean and healthy and also if you smoke. Sneezing may also indicate the need to clean the lungs.

The study of Ashwagandha is quite extensive because at some point, it heals the illness. Ashwagandha heals itching, but sometimes, you find that you itch but when you take Ashwagandha, it stops working. In a case like this, it may be that the skin lacks in Vitamin B, C or D or just lacks in all of the three.

The study of Ashwagandha also includes the understanding of how the herb works on its own, all its side effects and how the production of cortisol is regulated by this herb.

Why does the Cortisol level become low after showering or bathing? Could this be linked to a rapid sapping of white blood cells? The study of Ashwagandha, dry skin and Complete B complex, how does this work efficiently?

The lack of white blood cells in the body especially after shower may lead to severe itching that may be suicidal when not monitored and cared for.

Ashwagandha may cause the very same problem it cures, why and how can this be prevented? The daily importance of Vitamin C and its connection to the teeth, how? Vitamin C is needed to boost the production of Collagen. Collagen cells and tissues are needed in the teeth to keep them working at their best, so what is the importance of Ashwagandha and when is this herb needed the most for the teeth?

The teeth is one of the most complicated of all the body organs and Ashwagandha is one of its most powerful nutrient. This would make the study of the teeth and Ashwagandha a vital place to delve into.

Does the herbal intake of Ashwagandha ever subside especially in a world filled with free radicals and pollution?

How does the Ashwagandha work effectively with Resveratrol and Pycnogenol to reverse the ageing process?

How can Ashwagandha be taken when in syrup or powder form? How much will be effective and balanced for a new born baby entering the world of free radicals? Ashwagandha will be effective for a baby and throughout the adult life. Starting this herb early may strengthen the immune system and may possibly reduce the adverse effects of illness and ageing.

Ashwagandha as eye drops and as a nasal inhaler and spray, how possible? Ashwagandha clears the nasal digestive system and also keeps the mucuous membrane supple and in good condition.

Ashwagandha Shampoo, conditioner, mousse spray, serum, hair scalp, what can we gain from them? Ashwagandha restores hair color back to its originality and youth. Having the herb in just about everything may create a sensation such as a Cocoa Butter company!

How does Ashwagandha restore blocked ears? Ashwagandha may restore blocked ears when taken with Agnus Castus and tan tablets.

The study of Ashwagandha, dust mites, insect bites and allergy, how does the herb work? Ashwagandha can be taken with Quercetin, ginger root and Water Balance to treat an allergy such as sneezing when the flowers begin to pollinate.

The study of Ashwagandha and enzymes such as the pancreatic enzymes and the liver enzymes, how do they re-generate? Like the liver, can the breast tissues regenerate and regrow?

The study of Ashwagandha and depression: how does it control depression, anxiety and bi-polar disorder? The herb is taken with St John's Wort, Black Cohosh, Evening Primrose Oil and ginger root to control the depression and hyperactivity.

A look into the study of brain cells as we grow older but look younger. The brain cells sharpen the intellect and give knowledge, wisdom and power. The brain cells educate in the way of providing knowledge and wisdom for one's own protection and security. How does Ashwagandha increase the brain's memory and the brain's cells sharpness as ageing progresses?

What could be written fast and easy at an early age, may become something more thorough to write in many years time, which should be! At an early age, a person could think on the feet and write pages after pages even with new information and technology, the question is what can Ashwagandha and Resveratrol do, to compensate for this, as ageing progresses? With age comes wisdom, but the brain and its brain cells must be protected from Alzheimer's disease that may want to interfere.

How can we keep writing as if still in youth? How can we preserve the brain cells as if in youth? How can we keep the brain cells fresh, young and active as we celebrate the next birthday after another? We can keep it as just the next age only, but youth and agelessness eternally!

The combination of Ashwagandha and Devil's Claw cures a very bad migraine, what a deeper study could reveal?

Ashwagandha with Super Guarana and high dose of garlic oil prevents shingles, what is the complete herbal combination needed?

How about Ashwagandha facial scrub, body mud, foot butter cream, foot salts and foot cream? Ashwagandha softens the skin when taken on a semi high dose. It achieves similar youthful appearance for the skin which is normally associated with the intake of Pycnogenol and Turmeric.

The various reasons why we cough, what are they? It could be asthmatic, a stray food or drink, a weak lung or stomach disorder, or a weak cartilage. Whatever it is, how do we know which herb and cough mixture will cure the coughing?

Burdock, Ashwagandha, Slippery Elm, Acai Daily Cleanse and Sage Leaf relieve various cough problems that include lung disease and asthma, so, it is all about the herbal combination and the reason or reasons attributed to the coughing.

The study of Ashwagandha and Ginseng: which is stronger and what are their distinct values? Ashwagandha is reasonably the most powerful herb in the world, however, it does not necessarily mean that it has no competition or need for a combination. Siberian ginseng, Korean ginseng, Calcium, Magnesium, Sports Nutrition herbs, Complete B Complex and St John's Wort are just as powerful.

Ashwagandha delves deep into curing many illnesses and without much doubt, may be easily assumed as the missing TREE OF LIFE from the garden of god or garden of Eden.

The study and production of Ashwagandha hair oil, hair pomade, body oil, and aromatherapy oils. What ingredients will make this find, outstanding?

The study and the production of Ashwagandha mouth wash, souffle, lotions, creams, organic whitening creams and butter creams. What ingredients will make this study highly productive essentials?

The study and production of Ashwagandha body wash, body wax creams, exfoliating creams, what the best ingredients will be.

The vast study of Ashwagandha is essential because of its excellent quality and quantity in curing the mind, body and soul of uncertainty and failures.

The study of Ashwagandha is endless and unlimited and to study this herb is to gain a lot about its flawless endings and possible eternal qualities that may bring back to life the fountains of youth and the splendors of living longer than ever expected.

The study, the discovery, the possible and legal use of Ashwagandha in injection forms. Using Ashwagandha as an injection may however not be injected on its own. Ashwagandha may cause breathing problems at first, despite that fact that it also aids the breathing process.

In injection form, Ashwagandha should be used with Black Cohosh and ginger root. It can also be in the following forms:

Ashwagandha, ginger root and Vitamin C

Ashwagandha, ginger root and Black Cohosh

Ashwagandha, ginger root and Complete B complex although it could be used as Ashwagandha, Complete B complex and Brewer's yeast.

Ashwagandha, Aloe Vera Colon Cleanse, ginger root and some Calcium with Magnesium. This is one of the most powerful combination for resuscitating a Cardiac arrest patient or heart attack patient. Add Uva Ursi when appropriate but may not be used for more than seven days unless stated by Herbal Practitioner.

Ashwagandha, Calcium plus Magnesium, Water Balance and Aloe Vera Colon Cleanse pill

If there was no Ashwagandha immediately, then, L-5-Hydroxytryptophan would be ideal but must have ginger root as content in the injection.

It is also possible that when there are no Ashwagandha and L-5-Hydroxytryptophan available, Siberian Ginseng could be an alternative but must have ginger root and possibly, Calcium with Magnesium.

Ashwagandha, Hydrolysed Collagen, Spirulina, Oil of Peppermint, Cranberry, Complete B Complex, and Garlic Oil combination is especially useful to re-grow the teeth and repair broken teeth and damaged gums. The Spirulina energises the teeth sufficiently enough by producing tooth cells.

Ashwagandha, Ginger root, L-Tyrosine, Cranberry, L-Arginine, Garlic Oil, Brewer's Yeast, Complete B Complex, Calcium with Magnesium, Sage Leaf, Amino 1000, Cod Liver Oil and Evening Primrose Oil combination will increase the loss of bad fat, clear the throat, reduce infection, prevent anxiety attack, heal the vocals, repair the bronchial tube and the digestive system.

10. This method of resuscitating with herbs, minerals and vitamins are best achieved successfully, when done without adding synthetics and inorganics.

The study of Ashwagandha and IV drips to revive a patient in coma or on life support on an extensive level. Again, Ashwagandha should be given with a herb that aids breathing such as ginger root, Black Cohosh and Glucosamine Sulphate although with this Sulphate, it is best to add ginger root or Vitamin C.

Ashwagandha foods and soups, what are the best herbal mixes for this?

Can Ashwagandha leaves, be made into organic clothes, slippers and bags?

The study of Ashwagandha and Sun lotions, what can be done to preserve the skin especially when using the sauna?

The study of Ashwagandha as a milk shake, fruit drink and energy mineral water, what are the best combinations to preserve life?

Can Ashwagandha actually be packed as a salad, frozen vegetable and organic vegetable in the supermarkets?

CHAPTER FIFTY-TWO

ASHWAGANDHA AND PROBIOTIC ACIDOPHILUS

The Probiotic Acidophilus is beneficial for good bacteria. Taking it directly is suitable, but best taken with Ashwagandha in summer time for when treating a flu or a cold.

Probiotic Acidophilus is sensitive to heat and can be taken with Ashwagandha and Cod Liver Oil when in hot and tropical places.

Probiotic Acidophilus is normally kept in cool places or in the fridge because it may not work properly when in heated temperatures. There is Probiotic Acidophilus in Acai Daily Cleanse pill and it contains herbal mixes that aid better digestive system and good bacteria.

Taking Ashwagandha with Hydrolysed Collagen increases the hair growth.

Yogurt is also a unique way of enjoying a better digestive system and should be taken regularly.

CHAPTER FIFTY-THREE
AUTISM TREATMENT WITH HERBAL MEDICINE

Autism is a brain disorder particularly associated with children. This is a disturbing disorder, whereby a child lacks in major life expressions.

A child is said to be autistic if he or she is not responding properly to their family life and home lifestyle.

Autism is linked to epilepsy, asthma and a lot more complications.

Autism may be confusing at first, to diagnose perhaps because some kids prefer to be quiet. However a kid must always want to keep normality especially with their own family.

Autism should not be confused with a child's need to play or be reserved with strangers.

A child must be ready and excited to play games with his or her family, express deep emotions and show love to others in the household.

A child should be shown love, otherwise the child may withdraw and not necessarily be autistic as a result. It probably will be seen as a case of karma, where a child is going through a cause and effect lifestyle.

A child that is shown love and warmth would naturally respond. A child however may become quiet because he or she discerns that they are not loved or cared about. Most kids are friendly, as warmth is shown to them by members of their family.

THE CURE:
Ashwagandha is a powerful Indian herb and it regulates many problems for every age, because it heals the brain, the kidneys, calms a person, helps to express feelings and regulates the speech.

It also helps a child to sleep well through the nights.

However, because Ashwagandha is a very powerful herb, it should be recommended by a Herbal Practitioner perhaps in the form of syrup, powder or as indicated.

Ashwagandha is best taken with Natural Vitamin C, Evening Primrose Oil and Natural Vitamin B Complex with Vitamin B12.

Omega 3 is also very good.

Aloe Vera Colon Cleanse is also good for a child with gastro-intestinal disorder that may have being a complication from a brain disorder.

A child with oxidative stress disorder can have a nutrition that contains organic yogurts, organic cheese, organic milk, organic cornflakes.

DOSAGE FOR KIDS

There is a recommended dose for each age and depth of illness. It is best that each child take the dose recommended by their Herbal Practitioner at all times.

CHAPTER FIFTY-FOUR

THE STEADY EMBRACE OF HERBAL MEDICINE

INTRODUCTION

The future challenges for Health Care Management may include the steady embrace of **Herbal Medicine. The health society that we live in, accepts various medicine to survive, and for survival. There is the challenge in science. There is the need for a broader outlook in science and technology so that they can create space and time for herbal medicine.

BODY

In the *Life Extension Magazine LE Magazine January 2007 REPORT: Replenishing The Aging Body's Antioxidant Defenses* by Laurie Barclay, MD explains that when the cell's lipid membrane and DNA are guarded against age-related disease, it helps the body's natural immune system to fight off free radicals that may cause the aging process.

The body has its own natural antioxidant enzyme called the superoxide dismutase. The superoxide dismutase greatly reduces the oxidative stress that lead to cancer and many stressful problems of the organ especially the kidneys.

Although the body makes its own natural enzyme which is the superoxide dismutase that is found in the brain, it might be low. When the superoxide dismutase is low, the body is stressed, the skin becomes tense and may result in **eczema. Low superoxide dismutase in the brain and the body may also lead to high blood pressure and high blood sugar.

The Superoxide Dismutase is one of the main challenges of the future because it holds the key to a lot of youthfulness. It is in this section of the brain that the cells are kept young and strong even in old age.

The Superoxide Dismutase is the enzyme that regulates the body's DNA and prevents the cancer related problems from occurring. However, the challenge is on how to embrace the herbs, minerals and vitamins that help to alleviate the cancer cells that occur when the body is under great duress and stress.

The body is made up of macromolecules. According to the ^*UNM Biology Undergraduate Labs*, the "Biological Macromolecules are defined as large molecules made up of smaller organic molecules. There are four classes of macromolecules: carbohydrates, lipids, proteins and nucleic acids".

The four classes of macromolecules make up the strength and the elasticity of the skin and the body. It is why the body produces its own natural collagen, estrogen and testosterone to keep the body supple, soft and strong. But sometimes, free radicals slowly destroy the body and sag the skin. This lead to the aging effect because there is pollution everywhere: the electric wires emit radiation, pollution from transportation such as in cars, trains, and air planes emit heat that have free radicals in them.

This is where the herbal medicine become a challenge for the Health Care Management. **Herbs protect the internal and external organs of the body. Without the constant care of the skin, there will be no future.

There is the belief that there is no necessity for herbs and supplements. The need is much greater because of the replenishing of the skin and the organs daily. Food and salad are daily consumption and so is the need for herbs, vitamins and minerals to sustain.

The herbs need to be taken in the proper combination that would suit every **terminal illness and colds. Taking them daily will keep free radicals and pollution away.

The herbs are taken without the need of synthetic medicine nor do the herbs need to be re-mixed or added to inorganic chemicals to achieve a cure.

CONCLUSION

Herbs will always protect the human life. Herbs will prolong the human life in time and with time, but the right combination of herbs, minerals and vitamins must be achieved to attain an excellent Health Care Management.

The main herbs that are vital to regulating the superoxide dismutase are Resveratrol and the most powerful Indian herb, called the **Ashwagandha.

It is conclusive that the Serum Globulin of the body found in the liver will become one of the main health checks for the future. This is because it is in this **serum globulin that the health of the body is determined. This is where the body can tell if there is an infection in the body and how it can be healed and monitored immediately. A health check that has a level slightly above the required level, is as dangerous as a level that is much higher.

It is imperative that herbal medicine pursue the advanced method of treatment for all terminal illnesses via injections, serum, powder, syrup, tablets, capsules and drinks in the future, to ensure that speedy recoveries are placed for illnesses such as Cardiac arrest and **Diabetes Mellitus.

NOTES AND BIBLIOGRAPHY
FOOTNOTES & ENDNOTES:

*Life Extension-sponsored study #1. Changes in serum levels of superoxide dismutase and catalase in humans.

**Nona Jackson-Richie No. 13186. aka Miss Nona Adu reference to Diabetes Type II test results of HbA1c level –IFCC standardised mmol/mol unit between August 2011 and February 2013. Results now in remission. Remission since December 13, 2011.

^UNM Biology Undergraduate Labs: Biology Macromolecules; The University of New Mexico

CHAPTER FIFTY-FIVE
BUILD MUSCLE FAST WITH ASHWAGANDHA

Bodybuilding with Ashwagandha and Sports nutritional herbs reveal a lot of previously unknown facts about the herb. Ashwagandha is renowned for its powerful splendor when it comes to brightening the skin. Ashwagandha is the herb that turns an ageing skin into a flawless one. It removes all birth marks, scars, wounds.

It is a simply astonishing herb that is a must use. Ashwagandha is an Indian herb and it is nourishing for the hair. It grows the hair out extensively and voluminously to the extent that Ashwagandha's powerful work and attribute make it a Garden of Eden herb. Ashwagandha should be known as the TREE OF LIFE.

Build muscle fast with Ashwagandha and attain a strength, and back to life feeling. Ashwagandha is the herb that makes you feel eternal. It cures so much, it is virtually impossible to believe that it is not the TREE OF LIFE, that was said to have been washed away in the times of Noah and the Ark.

Build muscle fast with Ashwagandha to thrive better in life. It builds new tissues, new cells, rejuvenates, cleanses, sharpens the brain, regulates the adrenal glands from stress and provides life saving elements.

Ashwagandha is the natural life support of man. After Ashwagandha there is the Black Cohosh which is also eternal and serves as a natural life support machine.

Ashwagandha is so powerful it should not be used on its own. It regulates the diabetes to complete normality, it regulates the Sebum and the Serum Globulin.

If the Serum Globulin in the body is slightly higher or even much higher than it should, there is a problem in the system and that would mean that, there is an infection that may lead to cancer. This is where the high dose of Ashawagandha regulates the body system.

When taking Ashwagandha at all, there is an immediate and noticeable look about a person. They are calmer and more concise in thinking and in mental regulation. The level of most specimen tested from the body is suddenly normal. The normality is steady and may vary in each individual. In every individual, there is always a noticeable change whether it begins as a small change or a drastically good one.

Build muscle fast with Ashwagandha but make good sure that it is combined with the specified herbs, minerals and vitamins. There is hope in Ashwagandha herb for a life time restoration. Treating the body with detox also helps the herb to work faster and steadier while building the muscle that adds to the strength and endurance of this muscle, bone and body tissues.

Build muscle fast with Ashwagandha and enjoy a better liver. It works so well with the brain's neurotransmitter and the kidneys, to release stress and keep the body young and lively.

The possibility of Ashwagandha herb being regarded as the HERB OF ETERNITY is imminent. It needs to be discovered and re-discovered in many ways. It works best in each herb, with each herb and it nurses the skin back to youth.

Build muscle fast with Ashwagandha but take with Black Cohosh, Agnus Castus, Fenugreek and Evening Primrose oil to regulate the menstrual cycle.

Ashwagandha herb cleanses the skin from bites, stings and irritation. It is especially powerful in fighting virus and bacteria from terminal illnesses. Ashwagandha herb destroys virus by the aid of antibodies that are produced by the B cells or white blood cells. The antibodies or immunoglobulin detect and locate virus and bacteria inside of the body system and alert via itching or skin ailments.

Ashwagandha is extremely protein-friendly. With white cells, it fights virus and bacteria. But Ashwagandha does not fight on its own, it fights with Garlic Oil to destroy the viruses.

CHAPTER FIFTY-SIX
BUILD MUSCLE FAST WITH COD LIVER OIL

Bodybuilding is an essence in life. It keeps the body from stiffness especially in the neck and shoulders. Every day, you lift an item whether a teapot or a crane of fruits. The body is exerting itself and as it does that, it is usurping and absorbing. Build muscle fast in a profitable way for the body which needs a balanced source of protein.

The body is made up of protein. Protein are large molecules or macromolecules. There are four classes of macromolecules: protein, lipids, nucleic acids and carbohydrates. The large molecules are made up of smaller molecules.

The body needs fuel to keep warm and building muscle contributes to fat loss and a re-adjustment of the body for firmness and vigor.

The bodybuilding with cod liver oil is a major factor because it also contains vitamin A and vitamin D. The cod liver oil provides the essential oils that lubricate the organs and the muscle. The lubricating of the muscle is potential to the upkeep and natural maintenance of the body movements.

Cod liver oil is best taken for vision and alertness. Taking vitamin A directly and on its own may have side effects especially for someone who is not immediately aware of brain problems. The vitamin A may catapult or trigger a hidden problem that should have been detected and treated with more sensitivity.

Herbs, minerals and vitamins containing vitamin A are best such as Cod liver oil, Spirulina and Complete B Complex. Vitamin A on its own should be taken with caution and supervision.

Cod liver oil helps maintain the immune system and the muscle functions. Basically the body cannot be starved of essential oils because of their moisturizing effect inside of them. Cod liver oil keeps the skin moistened and soft but firm.

Build muscle fast with Cod liver oil and get the brain functioning properly. The eyelashes may get lengthier and voluminous when combined with herbs such as Milk Thistle. The essence of taking cod liver oil is to increase the use of good movement and ease of the muscle at any time in one's life time.

Build muscle fast with Cod liver oil and there is a higher concentration in the brain. The fainting and seizures are more likely to be reduced especially during strenuous activities. The eyes are healthier and produce brighter images.

Build muscle fast with Cod liver oil and protect yourself from a cardiovascular problem. The Cod liver oil provides nutritious food to the heart and as a result, the body can move normally without excessive need to lean on tables and walls. You can build muscle enough to have long walks and not have a cardiovascular problem.

Build muscle fast with Cod liver oil and relieve the brain of excess luggage, so to speak. The Cod liver oil is feeding the brain with essentials and the brain is feeling alive. The brain heals itself and increases in knowledge and ability to function.

Cod liver oil helps the brain to connect articulately with the heart. Circulation between the brain and the heart is credulous because Cod liver oil contains the powerful vitamin D that supplies the needed content to have a better and healthy heart.

Cod liver oil strengthens the heart. Like every herb, mineral and vitamin Cod liver oil should be taken with a herb that is recommended to increase strength especially when having extra activities such as the building of the muscle.

CHAPTER FIFTY-SEVEN

BUILD MUSCLE FAST WITH COMPLETE B COMPLEX

The Complete B complex <and Brewer's Yeast> is the bible of all terminal illnesses. But just not for terminal illnesses but for the prevention of diabetes and cancer. When the Complete B Complex is taken regularly, the risks of becoming ill are significantly reduced.

Complete B complex attacks the stress that come from workout, building muscle, typing, running and working generally. It conquers diabetes before it becomes destructive.

The fact that diabetes becomes destructive with complications once diagnosed or in the body, makes it fatal enough not to want to take a Vitamin B daily, to prevent this. You cannot ever stop taking Vitamin B or better known as Complete B Complex.

Build muscle fast with Complete B complex and enjoy the benefits that it gives. It contains Vitamin B12 a super active vitamin that takes control of stress. It controls stress that especially lead to diabetes, thereby reducing such chances of high blood sugar level.

Build muscle fast with Complete B complex and avoid the unnatural pressures of life. This vitamin must be taken daily. It is like the water we drink daily, like the food we eat daily.

A deficiency of this Complete B complex can be devastating. It can lead to low blood pressure, it can lead to Vitiligo that darkens and destroy the skin and the pigmentation.

Complete B complex contain vitamin B5 which is the pantothenic acid. It rectifies growth disorder and the thyroid disorder.

The vitamin B5 in Complete B complex, stabilizes the prostate gland and stimulates the adrenal glands.

Did you know that after treatment of the body system, there may come a time that chocolates may act as detoxifier!

The vitamin B5 in Complete B complex is responsible for the prevention of poison and itching, that may cause acne, tongue infections, shingles, dizzy spells and skin problems.

The vitamin B5 is also said to be "a morning after pill for gluten". That would mean that people who have celiac disease of the small intestines may be able to treat the disease and enjoy pizza and bread in moderation.

Celiac disease can have an irritating effect in a sufferer so taking Complete B complex with St John's Wort can heal and stabilize although the process of taking the combination may continue to be precise, that is, consistent in daily intake, due to oxidative stress problems related to environmental pollution.

Basically, building the muscle fast is more elaborate than it is giving merit for. It is a life changing episode and should be delved into carefully, and with much research.

Complete B complex contains Choline Bitartrate which is responsible for the transportation of fat and cholesterol in the body where it is needed. Choline Bitartrate is responsible for the production of acetylcholine, a neurotransmitter that regulates the muscle control in the body and when building the muscle.

Like every herb, mineral and vitamin there comes a time the body is over-saturated and needs to be detoxified. This regime provides balance with nourishment for the entire body system.

Complete B complex works at any time and at high dose for a terminal illness. It can completely regulate diabetes in a person. High dose which is supervised, along with the right herbal combination alleviate complications.

Build muscle fast and work out as normal. Gain the energy and the muscle strength that come with the intake of the herbal combination. This herb strengthens the muscles and restores torn muscles. The brain cells work well with the muscle and the understanding and sharpness of a person improves gradually.

Build muscle fast and feel the differences that ageing makes and bring with it. Ageing should only be remembered on every birthday while youth and the rejuvenation should be what is celebrated.

CHAPTER FIFTY-EIGHT

BUILD MUSCLE FAST WITH EVENING PRIMROSE OIL

Bodybuilding is a distinct way of building muscle in a body to attain higher strength. Prostaglandin controls the smooth muscle contraction and the blood pressure. The Prostaglandin can be found in the Evening Primrose oil which also contains the GLA, Gamma Linolenic acid that produces and regulates milk production in the human breast and body.

Build muscle fast with Evening Primrose Oil to reduce inflammatory of the muscle or bone. It heals the pain and protects the cells.

The Evening Primrose oil is especially useful for the health of the uterus, menstrual cramps, to prevent fibroids, to protect from sexually transmitted diseases and AIDS: autoimmune deficiency syndrome.

What are fibroids? Fibroids are growths of smooth muscle and fibroid tissue.

The Evening Primrose oil has therapeutic purposes that may relax the uterus and regulate menstrual pain and cycle. For a female who is building muscle, this method is a therapy that help to make life more comfortable.

Build muscle fast and improve the skin and body organs with Evening Primrose oil which is also known as Omega 6 or GLA. The GLA is converted to prostaglandins which is a hormone that is responsible for many functions in the body such as the maintenance of the cells of the joints.

Build muscle fast and regulate the blood to avoid blood clotting by taking the Evening Primrose oil regularly. It is also useful for the calmness of the mind.

Build muscle fast with Evening Primrose oil and relieve the skin of acne and eczema that may be side effects of the change of oil levels during new work outs.

Build muscle fast with Evening Primrose oil and avoid breast pain. With changes in the muscle and the body generally, there may be pain but taking the Evening Primrose oil bring comfort. The Evening Primrose oil promote healthy breast tissues.

Build muscle fast but prevent the side effects of having new exercises that may wake the muscles abruptly by taking the Evening Primrose Oil. Avoid the dreadful multiple sclerosis and headaches that may be possibilities of sudden changes to the internal organs and the brain.

The Evening Primrose oil promotes the absorption of iodine and is beneficial to the pituitary glands. Basically taking the herb is effective in promoting and healing, in many ways than one. It contains good fatty acids that keep the body in good shape. It also maintains the body temperature and relieves from high triglycerides that obstruct and interfere with blood flow especially during menstrual period.

The Evening Primrose oil can help reverse nerve damage from a terminal illness. The process may take from a year to three years, therefore best to take the fatty acid before having such an illness in the first place.

The Evening Primrose Oil treats rheumatoid arthritis and joint pain perhaps for its being very rich in fatty acids that keep the cells functional.

Build muscle fast with Evening Primrose oil and regulate the sebum that secretes excess oil when excess use of energy in the muscle is being built.

The Evening Primrose oil should be taken regularly when building the muscle, at fitness units, doing chores, brisk walking, whether playing golf or a sport, it is wise to take the Evening Primrose oil because of its many astonishing benefits to human survival.

It is as essential as having fresh vegetables daily. It is as essential as drinking water daily. The Evening Primrose is truly a masterpiece so to speak, when it comes to sharpening the intellect.

CHAPTER FIFTY-NINE

BUILD MUSCLE FAST WITH GLUCOSAMINE SULPHATE

Bodybuilding involves the understanding of the joints and the optic nerve. When there is a build of muscle in the body, there is also a fluid consumption. Fluid in the joint must be supple to maintain flexible movements and reduce pain.

Build muscle fast with Glucosamine Sulphate which is gathered or harvested from the shells of shellfish.

Glucosamine Sulphate has many functions for the body. It is useful for strengthening the optic nerve that captures real images. It maintains the fluids in the joints to prevent pain and injury especially after the build muscle fast regime.

Glucosamine Sulphate is also known to lower the blood pressure and blood sugar. It restores strength and energy to the joints and keeps the knees firmer.

Although Glucosamine Sulphate lowers blood sugar and blood pressure, it should be taken with the main herbs that are recommended such as Ashwagandha.

Build muscle fast and get the best movements you can achieve, for this is a brilliant idea when it comes to working and energy. A builder who climbs and paint walls needs scaffolding but he also needs to be empowered with working joints that can move as flexible as possible.

Build muscle fast and the way forward will be clearer and will also serve as an essential ingredient. Build the muscle fast for a good reason, so as to avoid crippling. Build muscle fast increases the chances of walking properly because the fluids in the joints are moistened and sufficient.

Build muscle fast and maintain good joints in older age is of significance because it also builds a stronger heart and better mind that thinks and flows with great ideas.

Build muscle fast and enjoy the privileges of moving about and even driving a car or a truck. Driving a vehicle can be tedious after a while but stability of the joint, and in the joint can be beneficial when Glucosamine Sulphate is consumed as required.

Build muscle fast can lead to a longer life without dependency. Build muscle fast can counteract problems accidental to old age. Walking should not have to become a burden as old age arrives. Flexibility especially of the knees and elbows are helpful with this mineral.

Build muscle fast and be fit. A better way to get up from a chair, stretch the legs, hold the legs high as you lay down and sit down without the painful and stressful effects. Glucosamine Sulphate when taken with other specified minerals and vitamins can alleviate a lot of difficulties that make life unnecessarily stressful and disturbing.

Day to day life can become complicated with teeth problems. The teeth gets easily stressed from extra activities but can be stress-free with Glucosamine Sulphate. The joints need to be pampered. After work outs, take the time to rinse the mouth with herbal mouth wash as this method de-stresses the gums and will reduce the need to have the tooth removed at any time.

Build muscle fast and be adaptable. Feel the need to stretch daily. This build of the muscle prolong the stamina and strength within the tendon, tissues and cartilage.

Build muscle fast to enhance the lifestyle. Your lifestyle is important especially if you are an athlete. Running, jumping and skipping are stretchy and consume essential oils from the joints and the muscle.

Build muscle fast and be able to fetch simple things. Either to reach up to a cabinet to get some salt or to open a window early in the morning, these things don't work by magic.

CHAPTER SIXTY

BUILD MUSCLE FAST WITH UVA URSI

Protein is the main body build of a human body. The body is made up of proteins, lipids, carbohydrates and nucleic acid. Uva Ursi is a tonic that should be taken as an herb for not more than seven days and every three months because of its strength and effect. However, there are other Uva Ursi herb content that are taken more often than Uva Ursi itself such as in Water Retention pills or Water Balance.

Uva Ursi is an astringent. It attacks wounds in other words, causing a major beginning of intense healing of skin wounds that may even be cancerous.

Build muscle fast with Uva Ursi and keep the Pancreas in good health. The Pancreas need to be cleansed quarterly to regulate the insulin production and keep the Pancreas in good insulin production.

Build muscle fast with Uva Ursi and protect the bladder from inflammation that results in Cystitis. When the muscle is built, there are toxins breaking out through the urinary tract and anal organ. At this time, there is a stronger need to cleanse and rinse and be watchful of symptoms.

Build muscle fast with Uva Ursi and keep the kidneys cleansed. The Uva Ursi is a tonic for the kidneys and removes excess sugar and toxins from the kidneys. The kidneys must be kept in balance to avoid an over filled organ that should be eliminating wastes.

It should remove wastes out of the body system and the Uva Ursi is one of the best tonics to ensure there are no accumulation of wastes in the kidney and urinary system. Wastes coming from the Pancreas must be flushed out of the system regularly to avoid cancer.

Build muscle fast without weakening the body organs. Taking Uva Ursi ensures that the kidneys, liver and the Pancreas are strengthened. Uva Ursi is a diuretic and it tones the walls of the Urethra and the urinary bladder.

Build muscle fast with Uva Ursi and have a more relaxed muscle and muscle tone. It relieves of pain that might have been precipitated from building new muscle.

Build muscle fast with Uva Ursi to strengthen the urinary tract and muscles, thus preventing bed wetting and other problems that may occur. A person who needs a catheter at nights may begin to discover that there is no necessity for it at some point because of better control of the urinary bladder.

Build muscle fast with Uva Ursi and avoid the dangers of been careless. Uva Ursi reduces bloating, it flushes out bad bacteria, it produces new and healthy cells. Uva Ursi constricts weak organs and wounds that may be as serious as amputation. It is a very powerful herb and begins the healing process instantly.

Build muscle fast with Uva Ursi and feel its strength as you work out and strengthen the organs that may sometimes be affected by new body development.

Bad fat that get stuck while being excreted out of the system may create more of a havoc if not washed out of the system. The bad fat contains bad bacteria and bacteria can easily accumulate when not treated.

Uva Ursi is also useful for when using the computer or electronic gadgets regularly. Typing daily and regularly can weaken the body organs when it is not nourished with the right tonic, herbs, vitamins and minerals.

Always care for the skin and the organs for they are being exerted to hard work daily.

CHAPTER SIXTY-ONE
BUILD MUSCLE FAST WITH VALERIAN ROOT

Bodybuilding is an important part of life. It should be taken seriously because of its adverse effect. While the muscle builds fast, it can also create damage. Taking the sedative, Valerian root at night may help alleviate damages to the muscle. Valerian root calms the central nervous system.

Athletes and people who do vigorous running would understand the consequences of carelessness. Some people run and then collapse at the goal post. It is important that the muscle is not stressed before starting such. Relax the muscle a few hours or through the night before taking on strenuous exercises to enjoy a more peaceful muscle build.

Build muscle fast with Valerian root because it relaxes the brain and reduces tension in the brain as well as headaches and migraines.

Build muscle fast with Valerian root after washing the hair with a mud content to reduce such chances of having a headache. Headaches are best treated when accompanied with shower caps on the head for a few hours or as required.

Build muscle fast with Valerian root and enjoy a good night's sleep before the hectic morning jog and work movements. Valerian root helps with insomnia and relaxes much of tension from various sources and from various reasons.

Build muscle fast with Valerian root so as to reduce stress that may occur from being too excited or being too excited or even carried away perhaps from a Wedding or a jet lag.

Build muscle fast with Valerian root to avoid epilepsy or fits which may occur during a change in the brain signal. The brain is very delicate and very sensitive. It could easily be deprived of oxygen and energy due to drastic changes in it.

Sensitivity must be given to the brain and the body when starting a new regime. A change in normal living in itself creates a problem that could be from mild to severe when not monitored carefully. Every little change in one's life demands a vitamin, herb or mineral to avoid deficiency that might be created from shock movements especially exercises.

Build muscle fast with Valerian root and avoid the pressures of anxiety. A person could become anxious for any number of reasons. It could be from preparation for an event, or preparation for an examination. Whatever may create such anxiety, take Valerian root as advised.

All sedatives should be taken with Ginger root, Black Cohosh, Vitamin C or Cod Liver oil for better breathing and circulation.

Valerian root is an antispasmodic which may help relax the digestive muscle and relax the gut as well as the intestines. It helps calm the irritable bowel area and improves the digestive tract, so as to increase in strength to break fat down into pieces.

Valerian root is unique for when having skin problems such as itching. The skin may have been injured or may be, in some form of pain. Valerian root is antispasmodic and helps to relieve the pain that may occur. It calms itching that may occur from an infection or from rashes on the skin.

Valerian root may heal and calm the skin itching and therefore may be recommended for other skin related ailments such as eczema and other skin problems that may accrue from itching.

Valerian root builds the muscle as it relaxes and eases pain. It builds the muscle fast by giving strength during relaxed periods especially when at sleep.

Valerian root builds the muscle while healing pain that may have been aggravated from heavy work out of the muscle.

Alternatively or additionally, taking a sports nutrition such as L-Glutamine aids the expansion of the blood vessels to allow proper circulation, maintain muscle mass and reduce bad fat.

CHAPTER SIXTY-TWO
BUILD MUSCLE FAST WITH YOGA

Yoga is the physical practice of the body and on the body to attain spirituality and peace of mind. The yoga practice which is of Indian originality, is designed to keep the mind at peace.

Build muscle fast with yoga and gain posture, revitalize the body fluids and especially maintain posture to avoid wobbling.

Build muscle fast with yoga and strengthen the build of the brain muscle and the nerve cells. Yoga helps with eye concentration, it helps to be conscious of the spiritual world and the spiritual realm.

Build muscle fast with yoga and build a stronger musculoskeletal body that helps with day to day movements, dancing and even singing and talking.

Sometimes the strength to speak is brief but regular yoga builds the affected muscle with the specific poses needed. Yoga should be combined with the right herbs to attain the supremacy an herb can give to the body.

Build muscle fast with yoga and strengthen the knees and the walking poses. This involves clever focusing such as THE STANDING BOW. This helps to reach a more focused and better life.

THE STANDING BOW: The mental faculties are sharpened and the mind is ready to move on gallantly. A stress-free achievement, it builds determination and power in the mind. It raises the hope and dreams to achieve and attain spirituality in a magnificent stage.

Yoga is to help you see beyond the mundane and the ordinary while you build the muscle fast. You can walk more steadily as it re-distributes fat all over the body and proportionately. The lungs expand as they should, to allow proper inhaling and exhaling.

Yoga may reduce cellulite although oiling the skin with Vaseline and herbal vein creams would complement the skin tone successfully.

Yoga tightens the skin and the elasticity of the skin. There is that firmer feeling attained while practicing various poses. The idea of practicing yoga is to attain a certain goal. A final goal may be achieved by reaching a obese-free state on the weight scale. Yet, a final goal in yoga would also mean continuity when ideal. The enjoyment of yoga can never perish or be diminished.

Build muscle fast with yoga and have a working digestive system although taking a herb such as St John's Wort help calm the nerves and digestive tract during the practice.

Build muscle fast with yoga by practicing the art of endurance and harmony. Yoga is like a teacher or a tutor, it teaches you the best ways to meditate and not lose balance.

It stimulates the brain's imagination. It takes you on a thinking pose and you are meditating naturally. You are accepting life as it is and floating as if over water but you must maintain the breathing process.

Build muscle fast with yoga to become the teacher yourself. Teach yourself how to be calm, how to be accepting, how to endure in a crisis. It is what bodybuilding is made up of.

Build muscle fast by meditating. Learn to sit on a yoga mat and upright, breathing in and out. The SITTING SIDE STRETCH is useful for building and stretching. Pose to attain good looking curves. This practice increases the strength of the sides of the body.

The SITTING SIDE STRETCH works for both sides to eliminate poisons. You feel the back stimulated and the hands toned. The hands work tediously and need to be exerted while building muscles in them. Move the hands to reach toes, back and forth and enjoy a healthier circulation.

CHAPTER SIXTY-THREE
HOW TO BUILD MUSCLE FAST WITH DEAD SEA MUD

Bodybuilding may usurp nutrients in the body during work outs and that is why there are herbal supplements. Detoxifying the body in Dead Sea mud, saps some nutrients from the body, but herbal supplements replenishes.

Building the muscle fast and at first, can cause tension in the bones and joints. Such tension can be eased by indulging the body with mud such as seaweed mud. After gently massaging the skin with mud generously, leave on the skin for thirty minutes to an hour.

Rinse off with warm water or have a shower with herbal bath & shower wash. Then wrap up with a towel. This regime should be done preferably at night or in a Spa Sanctuary. Making use of spa mud should be done quarterly or as desired.

Dead Sea black mud is high in salt and mineral content thus making it useful for the hydrating process. This eliminates toxins from the inner body and external skin.

The Dead Sea black mud does not necessarily heal all the illnesses of the world but it may maintain the skin's balance and texture and may help prevent diseases when taking with the right herbs.

The Dead Sea black mud helps to build muscle fast by reducing stress of the muscle thus, relaxing the skin and preparing the muscle for more energizing build.

Toxins are drawn out of the skin cells to rejuvenate the skin back to its youthful look and appearance. The elasticity is visible, nourishing and healthy in appearance. The skin is moist and fresh. The skin is less prone to infection and free radicals.

The Dead Sea black mud hydrates the scalp and for better results, always use a shower cap when having the treatment. The shower cap has many powerful uses such as for headaches and some mild migraine. However the shower cap should not be overly used for many hours to allow steam and fresh air into the hair and hair follicles.

How to build muscle fast with Dead Sea black mud is challenging when also applied to the hair scalp and the entire body. For the hair, cover with a shower cap for thirty minutes or as required. The hair follicles become healthier and this should allow the hair to grow better, fuller and longer.

On how to build muscle fast with Dead Sea black mud would be beneficial because it opens the pores to proper circulation. The muscle builds a healthier leaner self.

To build the muscle with mud is to be ready for more flexibility and steadier movement. The muscle build is to give a stress-free life and unburden the mind of unwanted problems.

Stress may have been caused from grief, pain, illness, a bad cold, over working and injury. The Dead Sea black mud provides the nutrients and benefits that are needed. Blood circulation is better and should function in a healthier, fresher way.

The Dead Sea black mud may help fight varicose veins and treat it. However, varicose vein may become a more tragic wound on the skin during a terminal illness and may lead to rapid cancer. It is best that varicose veins get treated immediately to avoid a more serious problem or even amputation, especially of the leg.

Varicose veins from stress or work outs should be treated with natural herbs such as the Varicose-Vein friendly St John's Wort that steadily blends the area back to skin texture. Normal flow of blood circulation is re-established and blood gets pumped to and from the heart as normal again to avoid a heart attack.

CHAPTER SIXTY-FOUR

HOW TO BUILD MUSCLE FAST WITH FENUGREEK

On how to build muscle fast is to be aware of other effects that should be monitored. When bodybuilding begins, the body may be exposed to high triglycerides which means that there is fat in the blood that should not be there and may cause a heart attack.

The building of the muscle fast is healthy only if the health check for high triglycerides are monitored. The triglyceride must not be higher than the good fat in the body system. Excess fat must be cleansed out of the blood system to allow proper flow to the blood and from the blood.

Heart attack and brain damage may occur when there is negligence. However, Fenugreek is an herbal plant that controls the cholesterol. It promotes healthy fat in the liver and removes bad fat that are known as the high triglycerides.

When bad fat blocks the blood circulation, there is insufficiency as to healthy circulation, and when there is insufficiency, there is a collapse in the body system.

There should be enough blood flowing into the brain because the bodybuilding work is consuming a lot of energy. Sufficient oxygen must be flowing to the brain to avoid such tragedies such as paralysis, stroke and heart problems.

Fenugreek helps the liver and the pancreas to break down the high triglycerides. It is possible that bad fat breaking out of the liver and pancreas enter the bloodstream but must be removed and regulated immediately with Fenugreek.

Checking the blood pressure regularly is essential to avoid an attack. On building muscle fast, there is the need to understand that high triglyceride could be an issue and taking Fenugreek stabilizes. Health checks done within a few days may give a high result when the Fenugreek is started.

However, it should begin to work at its best, within a week to a few weeks especially when taken with the right herbs.

Within a week or more, the Fenugreek should have absorbed into the system, creating more of a stability. The blood and urine test results should be reading with changes that are reasonable.

With such herbs, time is needed but the body is feeling the changes. The muscles are looking healthier and leaner. There is a freshness of the mind.

It is normal to make use of the bathroom frequently until the body starts to regulate.

Healthy eating does not mean strenuous dieting. There is plenty to eat but in moderation. Following the fat and sugar guidelines for your country is also a good way of setting the nutritious target for yourself.

The body needs enough fat and sugar, yet it also has a need to shed excess fat. There is a balance, the body needs fairness.

Phytoestrogens are in Fenugreek. The phytoestrogen works like estrogen and it is a vital component in fertility and milk production. The phytoestrogen is interesting because it is a nutrition that is needed when foods such as beans are not immediately available.

Fenugreek provides the phytoestrogens that are also rich in high fiber such as would be found in cereals, soybeans and beans. Fenugreek keeps both the internal and external organs rich and supple. You feel rich because it is a rich source of natural foods which is in the form of phytoestrogen.

Fenugreek stimulates the sweat production and prevents cancer in the body. This would mean that Fenugreek works well for both the male and the female reproductive organs. Fenugreek also prevents tumor and breast cancer. It may be best to take Fenugreek with Sage Leaf to ensure the stability while building muscle fast.

CHAPTER SIXTY-FIVE

HOW TO BUILD MUSCLE FAST WITH LEMON BALM

Bodybuilding gives the body flexibility. There is room for growth, there is space for breathing. On how to build the muscle has an important detail that guides through the lifespan. The detail is the virus and the bacteria in the body fat and fluids that are breaking down as the body builds.

The detail is vital to accomplishing and to survival. Lemon Balm is one of the biggest discoveries in the human history. But why? That would be because of its strength in destroying bacteria in the entire system.

Lemon Balm is one of the most powerful slimming herb in the world. Its recent discovery is astonishing because of its many qualities and capacity to conquer cancer and terminal illnesses. It heals from colds and flu. It heals the digestive system. It heals from nausea as it slims and flattens the tummy.

The lemon balm is the tummy tuck, and when taken with the right herbs, it works even faster. The ability of this herb to regulate the body system is unique. On high doses, it slims the body as fast and may act as a mild sedative.

The lemon balm therefore is recommended when building the muscle fast. This is a number one when it comes to slimming. It firms the tummy, it retains the natural shape and it cleanses the intestines of bad bacteria.

There are various herbs that work best with lemon balm. Lemon Balm and Aloe Vera Colon Cleanse may be best for the slimming and the anal cleansing.

Lemon Balm and Cranberry may be best for slimming and caring for the urinary tract duct. Lemon Balm may be mixed with various herbs to achieve one of the best results in the world.

On how to build muscle fast is to enjoy good bacteria while taking lemon balm. The herb extinguishes, in other words bad bacteria that may be destroying the eyes. It is also good for sore throats although should be combined with Burdock, Sports nutrition or Sage Leaf for best results.

On how to build muscle fast, there are factors to consider if you have skin disorders. Lemon Balm should be combined with the most powerful herb, I believe, in the world, which is Ashwagandha. This herb known as Ashwagandha is an Indian herb and it works with a lot of herbs.

The fiery combination of Ashwagandha and Lemon Balm destroys cancer and also help the body to enjoy the building of the muscle fast. The protein in the body is sustained and regulated.

On how to build muscle fast is a crucial time in a person's life and to avoid creating a toxic problem, the detoxifying of the digestive system and the body organs by the intake of Lemon Balm, is a discovery that is worth the note.

On how to build muscle fast with Lemon Balm is to be prepared for a new lifestyle. The lifestyle is so new, that caution must be taken by learning to be calm and relaxed. Watch this new lifestyle take up! What are the benefits and what are the self-conscious areas that should be heeded in time.

Building the muscle fast involves wanting to either look more masculine as to the male or more beautiful and feminine as to the female species.

Lemon Balm keeps the brain calm in a mild way. It may be taken in higher doses but need professional supervision just as working out needs a trainer to ensure that energy is not being overly consumed.

CHAPTER SIXTY-SIX

HOW TO BUILD MUSCLE FAST WITH PYCNOGENOL

To build muscle fast is to be ready to balance effectively. To build muscle fast can be achieved, but must be done with the correct supplements to avoid cancerous side effects.

To build muscle fast is to break the fat faster. The faster the fat in the body breaks, the higher the blood pressure might be, due to the sudden changes. To build muscle fast would mean changes in the cholesterol and because of the speed, there should be a balance.

How to build muscle fast is to weigh much in possibilities. A faster muscle needs sufficient protein. Natural protein drinks are recommended. Healthy foods are encouraged rather than diet. Organic and natural foods are healthy enough to avoid the compulsive necessity to dieting.

How to build the muscle can be done by HEAD TO FLOOR STRETCH in yoga. Always inhale as you exhale in this yoga practice. Doing THE COBRA would give strength to the shoulders and the hands when both palms are down. The chest should be erect, and head should be facing up in this posture.

How to build muscle fast should be done with care. Ensure that there are no ulcers on the skin so that the leg is circulating properly. It is easy to store wounds at this fast times and easy to be neglected because of the new look. Faster muscle build can be good, because negligence is avoided and risks are treated with utmost care.

Excess intake of protein drinks have side effects so make a daily plan of how to build muscle fast. Every day and by the morning, there is a change in this faster work outs. Note which days are faster, note which exercises and poses you did slimmed the body down at record time.

Note which dose of herbal supplement you took. Make a plan table that you can follow.

Pycnogenol works like a Botox injection when taken with the specific herbs. Taking Pycnogenol with Ashwagandha is one of life's fastest discoveries although both are the main ingredients. The process of building the muscle fast is beautiful and takes time and energy to get that far in good health.

On how to build muscle fast is to oil the body often in one day. The skin may be slightly more sensitive and may need thorough cleansing. Sugar scrub washes off oil sticking on the skin when drops of tea tree oil is added into the bucket of water.

On how to build muscle fast is to oil the body with Vaseline because it is a thick moisturizer. You can oil the body with Souffle and lotion. To oil the body with Vitamin E it is best to mix in some Vaseline or a thick moisturizer such as Natural Shea butter or Cocoa butter. This is to prevent the skin from the harshness of environmental pollution that leads to dermatitis.

On how to build muscle fast is to take Pycnogenol to increase the skin stability and elasticity, improve the hair growth and prevent blockages that may be associated with heavy fat loss. The muscle build is fast because of a motive to keep it on a lasting level. When the precautions are adhered to, the chances are that the muscle build does not need to slack and weaken with time.

On how to build muscle fast is to be weary of sunburn. The build of the muscle can be maintained in a sauna or in a hot environment. There is the need to make use of sun lotion at all times. Cod liver oil contains vitamin D that sustains good skin.

CHAPTER SIXTY-SEVEN
HOW TO BUILD MUSCLE FAST WITH ROYAL JELLY

Bodybuilding begins early, at least it should begin early to avoid the hindrances that come afterwards. Depending on the body's metabolism, the building of the muscle fast can vary.

To build the muscle fast could be best when stretching, and it could also be adequate as skipping routines daily for another. The royal jelly adequately ensures that the metabolism work at its best for every individual when taking with recommended herbs, vitamins and minerals.

On how to build muscle fast with royal jelly is favorable because royal jelly, which is extracted from bees, metabolizes the liver fat. It then contributes to the build of good muscle that shape dramatically.

Royal Jelly has a lot more functions and is beneficial to the body at any time. It should however be taken as acceptable to the body because of its strength and value. It may irritate the digestive tract that is new to it. It may cause nausea because of the breakdown of fat caused by building the muscle faster.

When taking the royal jelly, it may be best to take it with Lemon Balm, Super Lactase Enzyme, Full Digestive Enzyme or St John's Wort to prevent further irritation of the tract and to treat the digestive tract.

On how to build muscle fast and as the body fat begins to break faster to achieve faster muscle, there is the need to note the cholesterol levels.

The cholesterol levels may be affected by the rapid breakdown of fats and fluids. With the herbal intake, there should be a brain stability to avoid damage and mental problems.

Every individual may vary as the build in muscle gets faster and because of this speed, it is best to work out at one's one speed and at one's own strength. The importance of the build in muscle fast regime is to enjoy a new life and possibly a new lifestyle.

The building of the muscle is unique to each individual and to build muscle fast is to take a nap and perhaps, have a stop watch. Take note of yourself and daily strength. Drink because you want to. Have fresh drinks and mineral water, drinks that contain protein, drinks that contain vitamins and healthy drinks in general.

Chronic respiratory disorders may be a side effect of work outs, so why not take the right herb to prevent such disorders. Changes in the body mean breathing in a new way. To breathe in a healthier way, is to expand the lungs for its better breathing purposes.

The royal jelly increases the blood circulation and may be useful after strenuous work or after a jet lag because it stabilizes the liver. It increases the stamina and supports good physique. The royal jelly has a lot of functions. It energizes and restores the vision. The royal jelly brightens the vision especially on tedious days when the liver is so tired and exhausted.

The royal jelly acts as a tonic after the day's build of the muscle. It also softens the skin like Pycnogenol and vitamin E. It keeps the skin in bright condition and help it maintain its glow and color.

On how to build muscle fast is to create a breakdown of fluids that may need to be eliminated. The royal jelly may act as fast when digested during the weeks of the work outs but best taken with St John's Wort which destroys viruses in the body system.

CHAPTER SIXTY-EIGHT

HOW TO BUILD MUSCLE FAST WITH VITAMIN D

Bodybuilding encourages a feel good appearance. There is hope, there is attraction beaming in the heart. Building muscle can be for many reasons. If you are a singer, you want to be on stage and be healthy. You get fit and consume natural vitamin D.

Vitamin D contributes to the normal function of the body. It prevents scurvy looking skin. It absorbs calcium normally and contributes to the normal cell function of the nervous system.

On how to build muscle fast is by absorbing vitamin D. When the vitamin is taken, it prevents side effects from being in the sun constantly and promotes proper absorption.

Vitamin D carries a lot of weight because it is one of the main vitamins needed to sustain the body from terminal illnesses. The skin may lose its color entirely because of a lack of this vitamin.

Building the muscle fast may mean losing the vitamin D faster. Taking the vitamin D daily along with the faster work outs keep the color of the skin glowing. If vitamin D is lacking in the body, the organs may weaken, it may develop into pigmentation problems and tumors might occur.

Health checks evaluate the amount of vitamin D in the body and this must be at the normal level. Vitamin D contributes to the healthy growth in hair, giving the hair is color and keeping the hair follicles functional. Vitamin D may contribute to voluminous and lengthy hair when taking with recommended herbs.

How to build muscle fast with vitamin D contributes to the better function of the muscle. Vitamin D especially contributes to the healthier function of the bones. It prevents the bones from weakness. Strengthens the kidneys and the liver.

On how to build muscle fast is to understand how vitamin D works. The vitamin prevents the softening of the bones, a disease known as rickets. When the bones are weak, they cause the body to cripple. Sometimes excess work outs might affect the bones later on, in life. It is best to take the natural vitamin D daily and wisely.

The bones tend to weaken from vigorous exercise. To prevent diseases such as multiple sclerosis, there is the vitamin D. The symptoms are another way of taking care and having the necessary herbs and vitamins that make healthy.

Build the muscle fast but with vitamin D and ensure that the body does not lack in this vitamin at any time. A lack of vitamin D can be costly. A lack of vitamin D can cause the body to collapse, to wobble and then cause the need for a walking stick.

Preventive measures work best at the time of youth. Older age is not a prevention to vitamin D absorption although if the vitamin had not being taken from the early stages, absorption of it may be difficult. So, the recommendation could include a higher dose of vitamin D daily with other fast absorbing herbs, minerals and vitamins.

Older age does not end the building of muscle, it just means a different way of building the muscle is available and ready if followed appropriately.

On how to build muscle fast, there may be some wobbling as the body re-shapes, there may be some unsteady movement. Vitamin D with herbs such as Ashwagandha and vitamin C will help stabilize. The Ashwagandha should be taken at night times or as desired.

CHAPTER SIXTY-NINE

HOW TO BUILD MUSCLE FAST WITH ZINC AND HIGH FIBRE FOODS

Bodybuilding consumes a lot in the body and from the body. Starting a new work out may mean shock to a body getting ready to adapt. It could mean a blurred vision because new muscle also means a change in the vision. The eyes need to be cleansed and taken care of.

The taking of Zinc promotes growth in both kids and adults. Zinc gives vigor to the building of the muscle. It gives strength when working out. It sharpens the brain and keeps the eyes focused and attentive.

How to build muscle fast is healthier that way, but would be accompanied with the right regime that should include taking of Zinc and high fiber organic foods.

When building muscle fast, there is the need to have certain herbal knowledge. The Zinc repairs the pancreas. The Zinc produces insulin and regulates the pancreas especially in a person with Diabetes.

To avoid diabetes altogether, a balance in work out must be achieved. A high performing gymnasium equipment may build muscle fast but may also cause adverse effects on the body without the proper herbs and nutrition.

On how to build muscle fast involves the careful care of the ears. The removal of fat to avoid blockage and tinnitus which is the ringing of bells in the ears is critical to the stability of the brain. The muscle builds fast but it breaks fluids into areas that it should not. When building muscle fast, take fluid retention pills that regulate fat and fluids breaking out of the system.

Zinc also protects from benign prostatic hyperplasia, erectile dysfunction and infertility. For quality results, Zinc should be taken with Cranberry and St John's Wort.

To build muscle fast with Zinc is to be fitter and more resilient in many areas of life. Zinc is a very active metal and can be found in various herbs and vitamins.

On how to build muscle fast with high fiber foods is to be stronger and more coordinated. High fiber foods protect the colon. The foods protect from hemorrhoids. The hemorrhoids which are inflamed veins in the anal and lower rectum may cause severe irritation and more serious complications if not treated.

It is why high fiber foods are as important as taking herbs, vitamins and minerals. Inflamed veins have no place in the body. They only put more pressure in the body system and create a huge sense of discomfort.

There are many high fiber foods in the market. Sweet corn is a favorite but must be as soft as possible to avoid teeth problems. Beans and red beans are high in fiber and nourish the body. Brussels Sprout is healthy for the pancreas.

To build muscle fast also would mean healthy eating. Having boiled potatoes with cabbage is one of the most important nutritious dishes. Some have organic rice with fried snails and fresh organic vegetables. There is the organic bread with organic butter. Organic cornflakes with organic milk and natural brown sugar are also essentials and significant.

By the time you have the muscle build, you are noticing dramatic changes in your life especially when it is combined with the best in nutrition.

Some people prefer to grow their own foods and vegetables, because of the natural inclination and joy, that it brings to their lives. A purposeful life that is healthy is also a healthier, longer life that equalizes with peace of mind. Gardening is a culture in itself and growing your own food means the awareness of natural health and growth.

Zinc and Copper, work hand in hand and there is also copper and tyrosine in herbal tan tablets. Interestingly enough, tan tablets also heal the ears, prevent noises in the ears and may remove ear wax when taking with other appropriate herbs.

CHAPTER SEVENTY

HOW TO BUILD MUSCLE FAST WITH BLACK COHOSH AND DEAD SEA PRODUCTS

Bodybuilding involves various forms of movements that build the muscle faster. The muscle can be built faster by dynamic stretching. This is by a number of leg and hand movements to achieve the best goal.

To build muscle fast may involve THE JUMP in yoga basics. This practice rejuvenates the body and removes excess fat. As excess fat is being removed, black cohosh stabilizes the body system.

Stand with arms raised behind the head, bend your knees forward and jump as high. Jumping several times improve the breathing and keep the muscles energized.

To build muscle fast, practice various stretches that relax the mind and the body. Stand on the toes, have the hands on both sides of the hips; push a firm wall with both hands or put each leg on a firm table, one at a time.

To build muscle fast is to want to have intense work outs which would need plenty of drinks such as Aloe Vera drinks, orange drinks and natural yogurts.

Everything that is done should be well balanced with quality nutrition and adequate night sleep. Taking black cohosh contains essential oils that benefit and rejuvenates.

To build muscle fast, physical endurance is also vital. Avoid an anxious mind by breathing in and out regularly, and follow the ideal plan that is fast but steady.

To build muscle fast is to enjoy facial healthiness by masking the face with facial mud at least once a month. Spread the Dead Sea facial mud on the face for some thirty minutes and relax. Wash it off afterwards with warm water. The face is prepared for a better, healthier lifestyle. With the muscle build, comes a better facial structure that can fight back free radicals.

To build muscle fast is to enjoy a body ready to absorb healthy nutrients that maintain good fat. High fiber organic foods build muscle fast, organic milk is rich with content.

To build muscle fast, take the moment to breathe in and out daily. Make stretching a daily habit, tip toe if you can, and just learn to stand tall.

Using a Dead Sea product to wash away excess waste on the skin and body would also mean the need, to moisturize the skin in oils such as coconut oil. The body is delicate and the skin is accepting changes as long as it is done in balance.

Make time to use the Dead Sea body mud on the body and wait for half an hour or as desired. Wash off and do the method quarterly or as required. The mud detoxifies and removes the toxins that may have accumulated from the stress of building the muscle in a faster way and with a faster method.

Make time at least two times a night to have some Dead Sea bath salts in water or have a bath soak in warm water enriched with organic body wash.

To build muscle fast with black cohosh counteracts respiratory infections and improves the breathing daily. Breathing improves as speech improves too within time. It creates confidence and brilliance.

To want to build muscle fast is also educational when it is done wisely. Build the muscle in a shapely way that will make you proud and content. You are educating yourself and educating others when you build the right muscles. Making the effort regularly, protects and promote rejuvenation.

Build muscle that would blend with your face and your physique. Be yourself and learn more about yourself day after day.

CHAPTER SEVENTY-ONE
HOW TO BUILD MUSCLE FAST WITH VITAMIN E

Bodybuilding can be a time of resolution to meet a certain standard in muscle build. To build muscle is to understand the importance of bright skin with vitamin E.

Building muscle may slack the skin texture causing it to lose some or all of its elasticity. With vitamin E, brightness is restored and skin tear is reduced. The faster the muscle build, the weaker the skin may become thereby ensuring daily focus and sensitivity via the vitamin E.

To avoid the consequences of tearing the skin or developing shingles, vitamin E should be taken regularly. Getting the physique is fast enough, tearing the tendons is not a good idea.

To build the muscle fast on a PULL MORE equipment weighs on the body. It gives toned tummy and stronger muscles on the hands and shoulders. This method is one of the fastest work out equipment for building the muscle but it can also destroy brain cells when not nurtured with vitamin E.

The PULL MORE equipment could be at the gymnasium. It could be with a fishing equipment. A fishing equipment is a form of body building because the hands and shoulders are working and being exercised. Energy is being consumed whether the catch was a big fish or a small fish.

The PULL MORE regime, such as in pulling a rope or in pulling something, is a task, and a fast way in building the muscles. When something is pulled, strength is being exerted and the body is nourished with sufficient protein.

Vitamin E protects the body from oxidative stress that may come from pulling or dragging heavy items, from sweating while pulling, from breathing heavily and walking faster. The vitamin E protect the cells from excess sunlight, radiation and pollution.

Vitamin E protects the legs from blocked arteries and rescues the legs from pain. Running and pulling items may help shed fat that may also build the muscle, but vitamin E gives the legs the essential oils that it needs.

To build muscle fast is an achievement and proper care of the body should be noted from time to time. Toxins are shed with bad fat and eliminating bad fat is important, to avoid an illness. When toxins are shed with bad fat they are eliminated by the colon and the skin.

To build muscle fast is to wash the skin with organic soap and to help eliminate waste cells as they occur. When combined with the right herbs, it protects the brain cells and increases the concentration.

Sweat may cause itching and skin problems but taking vitamin E can counteract such irritation such as by having it with Garlic Oil.

To gain muscle fast is a marvelous period in time and when exercising on a rowing machine which is coordinated by pulling, always balance afterwards with vitamin E. This prevents a brain failure that may occur from the use of exertion on the hands and from muscles of the hands.

The rowing machine also works on the legs as you pull with the hands, back and forth. The buttocks get firmer and the body's need to build muscle is shaping well with the herbal intake of vitamin E.

On how to gain muscle fast is luxurious in its own way because it gives suppleness to the skin and emulsifies the inside of the body too. After a hard day's muscle build, try soaking the feet in a bowl of warm water with Dead Sea salts. The salts hydrate the feet.

A good combination of vitamin E, Pycnogenol and Ashwagandha brighten dull and saggy skin especially a skin that may have been destroyed from a terminal illness.

CHAPTER SEVENTY-TWO
HOW TO GAIN MUSCLE FAST WITH L-HYDROXYTRYPTOPHAN-5

To gain muscle is to want to regulate the neurotransmitter, Serotonin, in the brain with 5HTP. The L-Hydroxytryptophan-5 OR the 5HTP, is made from the amino acid called Tryptophan. The 5HTP may be found in Turkey and Chicken.

5HTP or L-Hydroxytryptophan-5 help build the muscle fast by raising the Serotonin levels. When the Serotonin level is high enough in the brain and the brain cells, it stabilizes the body especially when working out and doing stressful work.

On how to gain muscle fast with 5HTP is to want to strengthen the muscle and the brain cells so as to avoid a collapse of the body altogether. The body needs 5HTP which energizes the individual so as to have the quality energy to work, move about, walk and travel.

To gain muscle fast with 5HTP is to want to enjoy a better vision, think better and be versatile and active. The 5HTP is like the fuel in the car, and without the Serotonin in the brain there is no energy.

To gain muscle fast with 5HTP is to build the right muscle and shed the bad fat that may be interrupting the flow of proper circulation. 5HTP helps with good sleep and keeps the brain stress-free.

On how to gain muscle fast with 5HTP is to be able to breathe but must be taken with Ginger root or a BREATHING HERB that is, an herb that helps with breathing such as Black Cohosh.

To gain muscle fast with 5HTP is to gain energy for the fatigue body. It also sedates, so that it should be taken at night time. 5HTP may regulate diabetes on a higher dose. It may heal open wounds and may also be useful for cancer and terminal illnesses.

To gain muscle fast with 5HTP is to relieve one's self of migraine and headaches that may come along with heavy work outs and getting older. The muscle may wear out, thin out with age but the L-Hydroxytryptophan-5 or 5HTP, may help to keep the muscle in its youthful stage as it nourishes it without the stress.

Stress is the number one killer of all times. All terminal illnesses, cardiac arrests are all linked to stress. Without stress, there may never be a heart attack. Without stress there may be a reduction in terminal illnesses and all you have to worry about is the daily pollution and free radicals in the atmosphere.

Free radicals and pollution carry stress related illnesses and destroy the skin.

L-Hydroxytryptophan-5 prevents the degeneration of the brain cells that may lead to Paranoia Schizophrenia. The skin is burning fat and excess fat can cause Paranoia Schizophrenia when not addressed appropriately.

L-Hydroxytryptophan-5 should be taken with supervision, basically, like for any other herb. The L-Hydroxytryptophan-5 is from an African plant called Griffonia Simplicifolia.

Taking the 5HTP is a beginning to having balanced work outs and activities and the prevention of fainting and dizzy spells. While the L-Hydroxytryptophan-5 raises the Serotonin levels between the brain and the central nervous system, there is need for caution when taking the herb, particularly because it is a sedative.

A sedative of this nature regulates sleep, tension and anxiety but may sometimes cause breathlessness like every sedative normally should. A Herbal Practitioner may be consulted on herbal combination and the best way to take a sedative, that would also be combined with activities and work outs that help gain muscle.

CHAPTER SEVENTY-THREE

HOW TO GAIN MUSCLE FAST WITH AGNUS CASTUS

To gain muscle with Agnus Castus is one of those healthy ways that promote virtue and even chastity. Agnus Castus is an herb that produces the qualities expected of nutrition and adequacy. Gaining the right muscle is more of an achievement than a tragedy when taken with Agnus Castus.

The productivity achieved from taking Agnus Castus is quite relieving. It has so many benefits. It acts as a natural fertility drug when combined with the right herbs. As a result of its fruity, nutritious strength, it acts as a tonic and builds the muscle fast in productive ways.

To gain muscle with Agnus Castus is achieved by working out in moderation and with a plan that is not too difficult to adhere to.

To gain muscle fast involves making a plan that is more of accuracy and of readiness, rather than unstability that wobbles. When the plan is more of stable work outs, there is more of achievement in the routine and more of productivity.

Achieving a healthy routine as soon as it is established is best, to avoid fluctuation and a slack backs. Routine that is not achieving, may cause disinterest, however a steady routine that is building the muscle creates a more stylish route.

A stylish routine is building the muscle in similar styles and poses regardless, provided it is done regularly so as to steadily achieved. To move completely from a routine is to start afresh which shouldn't become a burden if the style becomes steady and achievable.

To gain muscle is to understand the highs and lows of various poses and the use of gym equipment. As the muscle builds, there is a point where certain regimes become more of a permanent style, say a habit.

However, on how to gain muscle fast, have a daily plan and when new routine poses and exercises are becoming productive, add them on, to each day that may be found appropriate.

On how to gain muscle fast is about wanting to try. Have the stamina to try and build. Have the stamina to focus and be confident.

To want to gain muscle fast is to gain a deeper look at the health of the internal organs and be keen on health checks that are regular.

How to gain muscle fast is about facts and truth. What are you able to do a day? What can be achieved today? How can I make this special routine work for me? Where am I? Where do I want to be?

Who am I doing this for? Am I posing and exercising for myself? Is there a special occasion on my mind? What are my goals? When is my deadline per pose and style? What position is best to place this yoga mat to enjoy the poses that are loved?

To gain muscle fast with Agnus Castus complements this gaining of the muscle. While gaining muscle, the body hormones are developing in a more productive way. The hormones feed the body and ensure that there are no toxins threatening the uterus.

Agnus Castus is useful for prevention of fibroid cysts that may have occurred from breakdown of fats that may not have been eliminated from the uterus area during exercise.

To gain muscle fast with Agnus Castus would be by taking herbal tea such as Cranberry tea with Agnus Castus tea at intervals. There are other herbal flavors so that after every work out, whether office work, a long stroll or trek, gardening, horse riding or long trip, you can always relax with a hot herbal tea.

CHAPTER SEVENTY-FOUR
HOW TO GAIN MUSCLE FAST WITH MUSIC AND DANCE

To gain muscle fast with music and dance is beneficial and healthy when done in moderation. Many Singers have been known to combine work out training with singing, and some dancing on stage. When you dance, you move the muscles, you move the body generally. Some dancing that involve the bending of the knees should strengthen the knee area including the bones and muscle.

To enjoy music and dance is to gain muscle in a way that will make you more comfortable, and ready to gain the needed strength. Music has been known to cheer up a dancer and activate the neurotransmitter in the brain to a sharper degree. It is why music is said to make a dancer spin happily. It is why music is said to make a singer much happier while singing. There is a special tone, a special tune in music and in every dance movements.

A little dance move, a little step and you get a little happier. How to gain muscle fast with music and dance is a balanced way of getting things in perspective.

Some kind of dancing may firm the neckline; some dance strengthen the belly and abdominal area. Some kind of dancing such as belly dancing is focused on achieving the best shape around the hips and belly area.

There is the ballet dancing that keep the legs balanced. Tip toeing teaches self-control and stabilizes the body in its own special way. Dancing helps to gain the needed muscle around the ankles, thus, exerting balance and steadiness.

How to gain muscle fast with music and dance can also be achieved by having a more permanent step routine that is practiced daily such as the Michael Jackson THRILLER routine. The dance steps are practiced by many and with a daily routine also comes a readiness to keep gaining the muscle.

You can also make your own dance step routine and in fact it is beneficial to make various step routines that you can practice when needed.

Perhaps you want to exercise your neck, you write out a dance routine that will help you firm the neck. Writing and making your own dance steps with music that you love encourage the necessity to want to gain muscle and keep healthy.

How to gain muscle fast with music and dance can help with breathing activities. Breathing in and out becomes more natural to the body system and there is the improvement in that.

The digestive tract and stomach need to take in the needed oxygen that gets transported to the brain. Breathing from the nose is a good way rather than breathing from the mouth too often. After dancing for even a few minutes, you feel yourself breathing in and out. It is a superb way of expanding the lungs and enjoying the lungs while at rest again.

You are helping yourself to breathe better when you tap the feet to a music you enjoy or when you are singing along. The mouth jaws are working out and so are the muscles.

How to gain muscle fast is astonishing when the rules are followed; however, there is no need to get excessively vigorous because as you dance frequently, the body's metabolism is adjusting.

How to gain muscle fast with music and dance is a way of establishing regularity. Having a dance routine regularly would also mean the metabolism is acknowledging the body's need to breakdown fats.

CHAPTER SEVENTY-FIVE

HOW TO GAIN MUSCLE FAST WITH SILICA

Silica is a mineral that strengthens the nails, that grows the hair and regulates the stomach acid with the aid of Betaine Hydrochloride. Silica also contains Calcium, Magnesium and Zinc.

How to gain muscle fast with Silica is by taking this mineral when it should be taken and as often as possible to strengthen the bones and prevent osteoporosis.

How to gain muscle fast with Silica is to want to keep the teeth firmer because gaining muscle can also wear the gum and the teeth, causing them to weaken.

The teeth has to be strong as the muscle is gained. There has to be a balance in strength and power.

Silica promotes collagen synthesis which would make it skin-friendly. Silica keeps the nails strong and firm.

To gain muscle fast is just about the same as the need to want to keep the bones stronger. Gaining muscle means gaining strength. They work hand in hand or the result could be fatal. Osteoporosis has to be prevented by taking Silica, to prevent a reduction of bone mass. The bone may start to diminish with time when it is not fed and nourished.

To gain muscle fast with Silica would mean the proper building and coordination of the muscle and body movement. The muscle may wobble if it is not receiving the herbal treatment for it. Boron is a mineral found in Silica and it provides muscle coordination.

On how to gain muscle fast with Silica is to get the balance between calcium and magnesium so that the body can be stable. Silica is the mineral that works with specified minerals to help the body make its collagen, which is an essential protein needed for the elasticity of the skin. Silica keeps the skin supple and soft and maintain its delicacy.

To gain muscle fast with Silica is to maintain skin texture and enjoy healthy nails. Sulfur is said to work well with Silica to give the body this sculptured grip that it needs. The body may withstand hard walks such as climbing hills and mountains, and the coming down a hill or a mountain.

On how to gain muscle fast with Silica may mean the enjoying of bike rides on hard surfaces, walking on mini-hills and bridges and having the strength to maintain ponds. Muscle gain can mean hiking on little hill trails.

Hiking in the forests can also be an absorbing experience. All these various ways of gaining muscle can also mean a diminishing in bone structure and may cause brittle.

On how to gain muscle could be by going fishing or kayaking. Rowing the boat is very exerting but maintains the muscle and gives it mass.

On how to gain muscle can be enjoyed from sport activities that are loved such as golfing. Golfing can increase the stamina but can also weaken the bones when the right minerals and herbs are not taken.

Playing tennis, exercises the hands and as the hands are used daily, the playing with the hands build flexibility and good movement coordination.

On how to gain muscle is to increase the strength of the eye muscle and vision. The Silica contributes to this effect. The Silica is also a recommendation when growing older as it also prevents yeast infection and contributes to estrogen production in the body.

On how to gain muscle and take Silica is a way of gaining muscle, however, care must be taken when taken Silica because excess intake may lead to vomiting and suffocation in the blood circulation.

CHAPTER SEVENTY-SIX
HOW TO GAIN MUSCLE WITH ACAI DAILY CLEANSE

To gain muscle is to gain strength and vitality. The muscle is being gained but it also needs relaxation. Valerian root is an herb that calms the muscle but it should be taken with Acai Daily Cleanse because gaining muscle also would mean, a change in the digestive system.

The digestive system affirms a change as the muscle is gained either by work outs, by taking herbs or by practicing yoga or karate. Fatty substances are breaking down and so are toxins. The toxins must be washed out of the system to prevent a re-circulation into the blood system.

Gaining the muscle is strengthened by taking herbs. The herbs help to maintain and prevent free radicals from pollution. Acai Daily Cleanse is useful for weight loss as it cleanses.

The Acai daily cleanse, balances the stomach acid and reduces bloating and regurgitation. Acai daily cleanse contain Bromelain which is a powerful digestive enzyme that absorbs and aids protein digestion.

The power to absorb and aid protein digestion is essential otherwise there will be an accumulation of toxins, and bad fat tissue in the colon that may lead to cancer and other terminal illness on a longer run when not taken care of.

The Bromelain is found in pineapple so that it makes pineapple a rich fruit to eat regularly. Slices of lemon are also purifying and can be added to daily water intake by having a slice or two in a glass of fresh water. A slice of lemon at meal time is healthy and improves the digestive system.

To gain muscle is to keep the bowels cleansed to avoid constipation. The acai daily cleanse contain Cascara Sagrada that eliminates waste from the colon. It also acts as a laxative.

Gain the muscle and enjoy good health by taking the herb and essential vitamins and minerals. Gain the muscle and eliminate bad fat. Cleanse the liver, the kidneys and the urinary tract with acai daily cleanse and cranberry.

The process of gaining the muscle that will not become accumulated with potential problems later in life is to blend in and be ready. Elimination and constipation are major problems to note in having changes in the body system.

On how to gain muscle is also a way to replenish the muscle fibre. The muscle fibre contributes to the strength of the body system. Too much fiber in the body causes problems so that the acai daily cleanse ensures that there is sufficiency and adequacy in the muscle and the body in general.

The acai daily cleanse acts as a tonic but best taken with Ashwagandha or L-5-Hydroxytryptophan to keep the dopamine levels balanced. Excess oil ebbing out of the body via the skin or the hair scalp may cause irrational behavior, irritation and severe itching. Taking either with the acai daily cleanse will not only help the muscle to gain strength and vitality but also control the sebaceous glands and regulate the oil control of the system.

To gain muscle is to wash the hair with organic shampoo and conditioner. There are various types of hair products. Hair mud exfoliates and removes toxins through the system.

Hair serum keeps the strength of the hair and keeps the hair from falling off. It also keeps the hair supple as it blossoms and may promote the hair growth when combined with the right herbs.

To gain muscle is exciting but a lot of hard work indeed.

With the acai daily cleanse is an excellent time to take sports nutrition such as L-Tyrosine, L-Glutathione and L-Glutamine to lose the weight and maintain muscle mass. The acai daily cleanse helps to clean out the toxins from the fat loss.

The L-Glutamine also strengthens the small intestines that aid healthy digestion of food.

CHAPTER SEVENTY-SEVEN
HOW TO GAIN MUSCLE WITH ASHWAGANDHA

Gaining the muscles that increase the stamina has to be balanced. That would mean that gaining the muscles to shed the bad fat in the body system has to be one of the ideal factors.

There are various ways of shedding the bad fat and that would be by detoxifying the body by the use of body mud. There are various types of body muds such as seaweed. The preparation of the body to detox the body creates an excitement for the opening of the pores so that they can begin to accept and adapt to this new breath of fresh air coming into the body system.

Then the muscles are prepared to start the herbal intake of herbs such as Ashwagandha. The body especially the skin must be strong. The skin must be tightened. The elasticity of the skin is tightened by Ashwagandha which must be taken with Vitamin C, Black Cohosh or Cod Liver Oil because of its high capacity.

Ashwagandha is one of the most powerful herbs on the planet. It has so many functions and it is a number one in bringing stress down. This herb is the type that heals, cures and a relief on an Island's journey until rescue arrives. It is that strong and recommended for all terminal illnesses. However the use of the herb has to be supervised because of its side effects.

As powerful as Ashwagandha is, it does not necessarily cleanse out toxins from the body. That would mean that the specific tonic and cleansers have to be in place to help keep the body healthy.

The Pancreas must be thoroughly cleanse with Uva Ursi every two to three months and with Uva Ursi; the Liver must be cleansed with Milk Thistle; the Urinary tract must be cleansed seven days of every month with Cranberry; the Kidneys must be cleansed with Ashwagandha, Water Balance and Cranberry; the breasts must be cleansed with Hydrolysed Collagen; the throat and thyroid glands must be cleansed with L-Tyrosine.

It is useful as a result, to gain strength and muscles. Gaining the appropriate muscles that is also healthy begins this way.

Ashwagandha is an adaptogenic herb and that would mean that it contributes to real energy, stamina and much strength. Gaining muscles also may increase anxiety and stress and the herb Ashwagandha regulates as it is taken.

To gain muscles is to rid chronic fatigue syndrome, ebb out bad fat, regulate blood pressure, regulate blood sugar, rid diabetes and live a normal life.

Yoga is incredible when it comes to gaining muscles. Simple basics in yoga strengthen the bones, the joints, giving the muscles sufficient movements to work better. By moving the body in flexible ways, the bad fat is slowly ebbing out to allow the muscles to rise in other words.

The bending, the kneeling, the placing of hands down while you kneel in yoga begins to steady the body. Yoga reduces wobbling in the body. Running, brisk walking, playing golf and walking around, increase the chances of gaining muscles.

With strength you want to look youthful, stay youthful and that is what the Ashwagandha does. Gain the right muscles and enjoy new cells. Gain the right muscles and enjoy peace of peace of mind. Gain the right muscles and build the capacity to move about, dance and play tennis. Working stress-free is a brilliant idea for you are now able to do as much as possible not as less as possible.

EFFECTS OF ASHWAGANDHA:

Ashwagandha may cause drowsiness and should be taken preferably in the evenings.

Ashwagandha should be taken with Agnus Castus to keep the menstrual cycle flowing.

Ashwagandha should be taken with Vitamin C to keep the system in good circulation so that the muscles can work and yet, not get stressed out. Vitamin C is a strong ne for efficient digestive system.

Ashwagandha should be taken with Black Cohosh to encourage better breathing because Ashwagandha acts as a sedative and it would be recommended that all sedatives be taken with a breathing capsule such as Black Cohosh, Vitamin C or Omega 3.

CHAPTER SEVENTY-EIGHT
HOW TO GAIN MUSCLE WITH BLACK COHOSH

Bodybuilding is important in day to day living. Stress can complicate matters. Getting older can create difficulties in work, in breathing and in sleeping.

On how to gain muscle may become tedious if you had not done that as early as teenage days. Sometimes, you are trying to gain muscle but with great difficulty. You need a greater sex drive. The need to be driven to get something better is a great start.

To gain muscle is to increase the estrogen and testosterone levels. The amount of estrogen or testosterone leaving the body during work out must be replenished to avoid complications such as cancer.

To gain muscle is to be stronger. Taking Black Cohosh to replenish balances both the estrogen and the testosterone levels in the body. The body gives the energy to gain muscle and it expects to be nourished in return.

To gain muscle and have black cohosh would mean that herbal intake of black cohosh breaks down the bad fat. The black cohosh increases the level of good fat in the body, thus encouraging proper breathing process.

To gain muscle is to control anxiety and restlessness. Bodybuilding is a life changing saga and should be treated with deeper care. It is the time where scars, acne and varicose veins may creep on to the skin because of the excess oil pouring out.

To gain muscle is to regulate the skin and the oil levels. The skin may appear dry, oily or normal but the fact that there is a regular work out with sweating taking effect in a body means awareness and weariness.

To gain muscle would need regular exfoliation, washing of the hair to prevent excess oil and to encourage fresh circulation through the pores and follicles.

To gain muscle is to be careful and have a daily plan. Note the changes in the body, the weight volume, the fat monitor, the weight loss, the height level, the skin color, the lightness or heaviness of the body.

To gain weight is to monitor the teeth and the changes in the throat and the neckline. The shoulders are changing and so will the comfort. The shoulders are either in pain or they are relaxed. The body needs essential oils to replace the oils leaving the body via the skin.

To gain weight is to be conscious of the reproductive organs. Black Cohosh regulates the ovaries that are also linked to a brain neurotransmitter. This transmitter works like a hormone. The estrogen is a hormone and it is produced in the ovaries. It is also produced in the fat cells and the adrenal glands.

The estrogen although produced in the ovaries is also linked to a neurotransmitter in the brain that controls the kidneys and the adrenal glands. By so doing, it regulates the kidneys and the adrenal glands from severe itching and cancer.

To gain weight is to regulate the estrogen in the body which is one of the most important hormone in the body system. Its production in the body in a steady way reduces stress exceedingly.

On how to gain muscle is to ensure that the hormones in the body are not being sapped excessively by extreme work outs that lead to a downfall of the organs in general.

On how to gain muscle is to be aware of the estrogen's connection to the brain and the kidneys. Estrogen has a lot of functions in the body.

CHAPTER SEVENTY-NINE
HOW TO GAIN MUSCLE WITH CHROMIUM PICOLINATE

Bodybuilding increases the strength of the muscles in the body especially in the arms and the legs. The joints become more supple and flexible thus, giving the body an increase in good circulation.

Gaining muscle can be done by working out at the gymnasium but may decrease the strength in the body as time goes by. This is why Chromium Picolinate is recommended when working out.

Chromium Picolinate is a nutritional supplement that is needed in the body but in small amounts. It gives the body the muscle mass that it needs. It also ebbs out the bad fat as it increases muscle mass.

Chromium Picolinate, like all herbs and minerals, it would be taken with the needed herbs to ensure proper function and good health in the body. Chromium Picolinate maintains the bodybuilding effect and nourishes the blood system.

Chromium Picolinate helps maintain the good condition of a body that is gaining muscle, it helps maintain the blood pressure and blood sugar.

After a hard day, Chromium Picolinate relaxes the muscle as it gains strength. Stress is a daily occurrence in life, working out is work in itself and may even tear muscles. Taking the Chromium Picolinate gives more of an assurance to the body muscles than not taking it at all.

The Chromium Picolinate removes metals and toxins from the body system. It also removes mercury that may have been digested while eating, if there is a mercury filled metal inside the teeth.

Gaining muscles also means having the need for energy. Moving about on a daily basis is so stressful it can cause the blood sugar to rise. It can cause blood pressure too. The Chromium Picolinate regulates the blood pressure, blood sugar and maintains the insulin in the body system to avoid any type of diabetes.

STRONG EFFECTS TO GAIN MUSCLE

Take Chromium Picolinate as recommended

Take Chromium Picolinate with herbs that maintain the sugar levels such as Brewer's Yeast. Brewer's Yeast contains some Chromium.

When working out on a Close-Grip bench press or a gym equipment, ensure that it is done in moderation as the Chromium Picolinate help the body to gain muscle.

Taking excess Chromium Picolinate may cause damage so that it is taken in small doses. It would also be best to detox as often as possible. Milk Thistle is best for the liver and may counteract a side effect that may be cause by taking Chromium Picolinate. However Milk Thistle cannot be taken on its own.

Gaining muscle may help to increase the metabolism and thus, remove the bad fat that may be blocking the arteries or the walls of the arteries. As the fat is removed, blood circulation increases to and from the heart. The leg circulation is also maintained and energy flow increases.

Gaining muscle and taking Chromium Picolinate increases the eye vision. There is more of focus and attention. The mind is thinking clearly, there is better concentration.

Gaining muscle means power, strength, vigor, thereby indicating a need to relax. There is need for rest and ample time must be given to relax, get enough rest, get a good night's sleep and get ready by the morning.

Gaining muscle may include the taking of an herbal sedative at nights to help relax the muscles the body is gaining. Valerian root is a good herb that calms the body muscle.

CHAPTER EIGHTY
HOW TO GAIN MUSCLE WITH GINSENG

Bodybuilding is no doubt a good way of strengthening the muscle. During this time that the body is increasing in muscle building, the fat loss is giving way to something much better.

There are many ways of improving the muscle strength. Weight lifting is said to be one of the favorites but it has to be maintained. Taking protein drinks and milk shakes are part of the gaining of the muscle but in moderation.

Yoga has minimal side effects. Yoga trims the body and increases the muscle gain. However there is always the need to balance work of any nature with energy. This is why Ginseng helps in the concentration and stamina of a bodybuilder.

Breathing with the arms is a yoga practice. You sit on the heels with the hands under the chin, then toss the head backwards a little. Inhaling and exhaling increases the strength of the tummy muscles and freshness is inculcated.

This breathing technique is helpful for a person who sometimes may have difficulty in breathing. This is a singer's dream although a singer has to take Ashwagandha to stabilize the vocal cords.

Ginseng helps to gain muscle and it also helps to increase the stamina of a person especially after an illness. Ginseng may heal symptoms of an illness especially when combined with other herbs. It improves the blood pressure and expands the lung capacity.

Ginseng may improve the brain function where dizziness and fainting are concerned. It helps a brain to be energized and reduces the symptoms that may occur from new muscle in the entire body system.

On how to gain muscle, there is also a yoga pose that is called SIDE STRETCH. Stand with legs apart, hands stretched on both sides, then toss the chest forward a little so that the spinal cord can ooze the stress out. Gain muscle by doing this when you are able or as advised.

For every stretch there is an amount of sweat leaving the body. There is energy leaving the body and there is energy needed to make up for it. Fluids are essential to replenish the body system of loss of sweat and to prevent dehydration.

On how to gain muscle, there is that need to hydrate the body system. Exfoliate the skin regularly to prevent dead cells on the surface of the skin from staying on. This may cause eczema and other skin problems. Cleansing is essential and trimming properly is appropriate at this time.

Gain muscle to remove bad fat not elevate such. Aloe Vera Colon Cleanse removes the wastes from the body system, the colon, the rectum and the appendix. When the body moves from doing the exercise, it is also breaking down fats via the bile duct. The small intestines get ready to breakdown the foods and fat from the bile processing to the large intestines.

It is important that the body is strong enough to move food and fat as the breakdown occurs, from each organ to another and this is where Ginseng shows its powerful capacity to move successfully. Strength is always needed for the body's digestion otherwise it becomes slow and toxins begin to harbor in the intestines which may lead to cancer and other illnesses.

Ginseng also empowers the intestines so that they have such capacity to continue to work and flow without leaving bad fat, toxins in the artery walls, tissues or muscle fibre walls.

CHAPTER EIGHTY-ONE
HOW TO GAIN MUSCLE WITH HYDROLYSED COLLAGEN

How to gain muscle with Hydrolysed Collagen is quite a healthy process because of its ability to cleanse via the lymphatic drainage system. This particular combination of amino acids to make collagen is especially useful to lean muscle, firm neck, flat belly and lymphatic drainage of the breasts from breast tumors.

To gain muscle is to rebuild the organs. The Hydrolysed Collagen is so called because it gets soaked and dehydrated to allow easy passage for the amino acids in the blood stream. Hydrolysed Collagen is made from bovine bone and cartilage. Hydrolysed Collagen is preferred to Collagen as a result because of its easy flow of the amino acids into the blood stream.

To gain muscle involves a lot of health watch. There is the importance of building the organs, the teeth, making them stronger by Hydrolysed Collagen. There is the necessity in life of repairing the bone structure, the knee joints, the neck and possible hair growth. The eyebrows become hairy, the eyelashes become fuller with hair.

Hydrolysed Collagen is so useful when gaining muscle because it works on bad fat, tumor in the body especially breast tumor and when combined with Lemon Balm and St John's Wort it may remove breast tumor completely and protect the breasts from excess fluids and fatty tissues that shouldn't be there. Fenugreek is also a vital herb for the nourishment of both the male and female breasts.

Hydrolysed Collagen increases the strength of the bones so that the power to walk, run, jump, skip and dance are increased. It is a vital component in increasing the bone structure, the structure of the face, the shape of the body and reduces the chances of osteoporosis and osteoarthritis.

To gain muscle is to be above average when combined with the specific herbs. When you gain muscle you are shedding fat, you are losing weight, you are shedding fluids and sometimes the right fluids may leave the body. Replenishing is effective and Hydrolysed

Collagen stimulates and nourishes as it drains toxins out of the body system.

Gain the muscle but not lose a tooth is essential because gaining muscle can also lead to deterioration and weakness of the body. The muscles get tired and need food. The Hydrolysed Collagen is the food, it firms the neck, give it back its youthfulness. The bones of the neck straighten and stay firm as older age arrives but there is strength and there is also the possibility of a reversal in old age.

The firmness of the neck is of particular interest because it is where the significance of ageing is held high. Age should no longer be a problem as time goes by because of this discovery in Hydrolysed Collagen that firms the neck and the belly. The muscle is toned, elasticity makes the tummy firmer, stronger and better. Walking improves in older age and joining in simple activities should make life more bearable rather than a sentence.

To gain muscle is to be alert to minor problems. A minor problem can easily become a major problem so that care and health checks should be made as soon as they can be done. The skin is supple, smooth and the cells accept these changes because Hydrolysed Collagen helps to maintain youth and beautiful skin.

To gain muscle is to look leaner, appear leaner, with good fat in the body for warmth and suppleness of the bones and to the bones. However there is the need to be sure that it is good fat that runs in the body to reduce an increase in cholesterol levels.

CHAPTER EIGHTY-TWO

HOW TO GAIN MUSCLE AND ORGANIC BOTOX-LIKE CREAMS

Bodybuilding is the essence of life in so many ways. The body is embracing protein and in balanced ways that is refreshing. The bodybuilding encourages shape value and trim value. The enhancing of the body to build and not to be obese.

On how to gain muscle involves the skin value. It involves loving the skin and maintaining it. The gaining of muscle is also the removal of dead cells that must be cleanse to avoid apoptosis.

On how to gain muscles and stabilize protein in the body involves the use of herbal and organic creams that re-vitalize the skin.

On how to gain muscles involves the moisturizing of the skin to attain restoration. Aloe Vera is popular for cream use or herbal intake. It has fulfilling uses when combined well. Most organic creams have been well combined with the ingredients that are needed to sustain ailing and ageing skin.

The need to use such organic creams cannot be over-emphasized when it comes to gaining the muscle and working the body. A gymnasium equipment is such that anyone and everyone makes use of it daily. It is taken care of by cleaning and with cleaning detergents but somehow, you find that the need to keep hygienic in one's own right is crucial.

Dependency is not an option when gaining muscle at a gym or public place. The resistance of the body is going through major changes. There is that need to take anti-oxidants such as Vitamin C and these herbs and vitamins must not be synthetic to keep them working at their very best. Inorganic chemicals do not agree with nature.

Gaining the muscle and the body's new resistance has to be monitored. The body is being interrupted, being disturbed and needs full attention. The organic creams contain natural chemicals such as Lemon that hydrate and moisturize the skin day after day.

The skin works best when asleep in the night and there is a noticeable appearance of beauty in the mornings when oiled on the skin daily.

The creams are like natural Botox. The creams contain various ingredients that also slim and trim the body to shape. The cream may brighten a skin, it may add gloss to a dull skin. It depends on the type of skin. The oily skin, the dry skin and the normal skin all need to be moisturized daily.

Moisturizers that are not organic and natural may prevent proper metabolizing of the liver. There is the double strength Aloe Vera with Cocoa butter and Shea butter.

This type of organic cream works so well on the skin, it may also act as the astringent and antiseptic to wounds that may be as serious as amputation.

The organic creams may contain Uva Ursi from natural bearberry and can treat such bad wounds or eczema. Wounds that may have come from a complication during the work out or during an illness.

Taking an herbal supplement along with using these life-saving creams maintain a calmness and longevity perhaps never before visualized.

On how to gain muscle creates a perplexity for a person who is starting out on this adventure to gain muscle. This must be done properly with a proper plan and foundation to avoid such risks as cancer and illnesses.

On gaining muscle there is that need to ensure that no part of the skin is being torn or affected at such a time.

This botox injection is made of ingredients such as tan tablets, pycnogenol, vitamin E, ashwagandha, sports nutrition such as L-Glutathione and resveratrol. This is best with herba whitening creams, tea tree lotions, cocoa butter, shea butter and vitamin E butter.

CHAPTER EIGHTY-THREE
HOW TO GAIN MUSCLE WITH RESVERATROL

Bodybuilding with herbs make it more enjoyable and with the combination, there may be possibilities of age reversal. The resveratrol is an herb that keeps cells youthful. This herb works at its very best when combined with the specific herbs.

The resveratrol keeps the muscles and body working, whether you are having a drink of protein milk shake or you are jogging or running, the herb keeps the cells fresh and new. The resveratrol protects the cells from ageing and from cancer.

How to gain muscle with resveratrol is by taking the herb as recommended to keep it working faithfully. The resveratrol is said to be from a Japanese Knotweed extract.

Resveratrol has been said to contain longer life prosperity which is not too far-fetched when the right combination with other herbs is eventually found and manufactured.

Resveratrol contributes to the cell production, it balances the Super-Oxide neurotransmitter that regulates the brain's neurotransmitter and the kidneys.

Resveratrol regulates so that it may be useful for brain protection from Alzheimer's and diseases. It regulates the blood sugar before or after diabetes and may contribute to the repair of the Pancreas.

The possibility of Resveratrol and Zinc with copper may repair the Pancreas with time for a diabetic. It can also brighten the vision and repair the eyes but with time and in time.

How to gain muscle with Resveratrol works best with Lemon Balm, Aloe Vera Colon Cleanse and Cranberry to increase the best chances of a younger, better look. Taking the herbal combination will increase the blood flow and prevent blood clot. It will also help prevent blood platelets from sticking together to cause a cardiac arrest.

Resveratrol lowers the cholesterol and may increase good fat when taking with Lemon Balm and Black Cohosh. Taking organic yogurt, frozen yogurt may help fight bad bacteria and protect the gastrointestinal system.

How to gain muscle is by maintaining these steps to get a good shape, trim better and maintain a more youthful appearance.

How to gain muscle and enjoy it, would include having fresh salads in meals, fresh vegetables such as Brussels Sprout, Cabbage, Green Lettuce, Broccoli and Spinach.

How to gain muscle and detoxifying by eating Spinach is another healthy way of promoting one's very own muscle.

How to gain muscle with Resveratrol balances the health of the heart and the cells are more likely to produce new and youthful cells that begin to reflect on the skin. It is an important attribute to obtainable skin that is healthy and clear.

Having red grapes and blueberries is another way of keeping the skin flawless and youthful. Resveratrol may firm the bones and knees. It also may keep the legs in good condition.

Resveratrol may contain anti-stress ingredients but best to have it with Sage Leaf, L-5-Hydroxytryptophan or Ashwagandha at night time.

Resveratrol may build the muscle fast when taking with St John's Wort. The muscle mass with good fat is enriched with the herbal intake and digestion of Resveratrol combined with St John's Wort and Oil of Peppermint.

The soothing factor in Oil of Peppermint works with Resveratrol to flush out constipation. It is about the enjoyment of building the muscle, gaining the muscle mass that is needed and utilizing it as desired.

This herbs maintain this desire and condition the desire to build muscle fast but in the right way that will have no regrets or side effects later.

CHAPTER EIGHTY-FOUR
HOW TO GAIN MUSCLE WITH SAGE LEAF

To gain distinct muscle of the body, there is that need to take protein drinks, protein milk shakes, get the best in exercises and lift heavy weight equipment but sometimes gaining muscle doesn't have to be that tedious.

Bodybuilding is exciting when it can be maintained, but as older age begins to creep in, there is the need to maintain the strength that has been acquired when in tender years.

The herb known as the Sage Leaf is a highly recommended ideal. It has so many qualities inside of it. It keeps the skin's elasticity tighter and youthful as time and age arrive. The muscle gained is protected by proteins found in Sage Leaf. The skin looks fresher and older age becomes a name only.

Gaining the muscle can also be achieved by the Basic Yoga One-arm Balance. This is done carefully to avoid injury and starting this out might need the help of a trainer, if you are not familiar with how this works.

Gaining muscle with Sage Leaf can improve sleep and rest. It can improve calmness and take the anxiety away. It can increase the hair of the head and keep it in its natural color.

When gaining muscle you are also stressing, so there is that need to reduce anxiety and enjoy the fruitages that may be derived from extra strength and vitality.

Gaining muscle with Sage Leaf reduces tear in the arteries, increases the strength of the veins. For a bodybuilder, there are sometimes drawbacks such as coughs, sore throats and side effects when increasing the stamina.

The body is adapting to a new body and may sometimes have to be in some pain.

Gaining muscle with Sage Leaf increases the strength of the nervous system. It keeps the body protein fresh, supple and relaxed. Sage Leaf has a calming effect and for that reason, the cells of the body system are nourished in calmness and as it embraces this new body it is being created into.

Gaining muscle is an important time in the life of a bodybuilder. With a new body and shape comes new responsibilities such as ensuring that the mental stability is not deteriorating. A new body means changes and new responses in the brain and that would mean caution and care.

Gaining muscle could lead to various ailments within time but to avoid such side effects, it is best to take Sage Leaf in combination with recommended herbs. Having a natural or organic milk shake from time to time should be helpful.

Gaining muscle could cause a cold or a cough. It could cause joint pain because of various changes and movements. The circulation is being shocked into a new lifestyle, a new vision, a new style of walking and a new step. Every step that is taken is new, the body is becoming sensitive but must be regulated as it gains muscle, strength, energy and power.

Gaining muscle means the shedding of oil and the skin is having more dead cells to possibly shed. This is the time where the body is being watched for symptoms of ailments. When oil is being emitted from the skin, it must be regulated with Sage Leaf. There are other herbs that are useful such as Turmeric.

Gaining muscle is a special time period and with such times come the focus to take caution, take regular health check and study the body effectively.

CHAPTER EIGHTY-FIVE
HOW TO GAIN MUSCLE WITH SPIRULINA

On how to gain muscle is to be much stronger. Bones become stronger by every next birthday. This is because Spirulina has twenty six times more of Calcium. Spirulina repairs cells, it gives the teeth new cells. With Spirulina there is no actual need to fill the tooth with mercury and metal. It does it all provided it is combined with the right herbs.

On how to build the body is to be motivated to gain strength. Become super active and enjoy the body's movement without pain and aches. Spirulina contains protein and rejuvenates the cells. There is growth and the muscle builds.

On how to gain muscle is to reduce the bad cholesterol in the body. Spirulina reduces bad cholesterol and promotes the good fat. It stimulates the digestive tract so as to avoid bad bacteria.

On how to gain muscle is to take a regular supply of Spirulina. It is excellent for good eye vision and may be combined with the right herbs such as Complete B Complex. This depends on the strength of the body.

A weak body would need the combination and a stronger body may do well with just the Spirulina as it contains Vitamin B12 and vitamins. Spirulina is the highest source of vitamin B12, however.

On how to gain muscle is to protect the arteries. The Spirulina rids the body of toxins, infections and cardiovascular diseases. The Spirulina is also known as the richest source of food for the eyes. The skin needs to be cleansed as well as the digestive system.

On how to gain the muscle is to build the muscle mass. Build the right body mass so as to stay healthy. Spirulina is a blue-green algae that can be found in lakes and ponds.

Spirulina contains Iron and Vitamin K and these are essential to the gaining of the muscle without falling apart. The body must be nourished to avoid a collapse of during work outs. The scalp must be firm not wobbling. The knees must be firm and not wobbling. Spirulina gives the strength and tonic when it is needed the most.

Spirulina benefits the digestive system with good bacteria that prevents indigestion, vomiting and regurgitating. It also prevents the irritation of the digestive tract especially when combined with Lemon Balm.

On how to gain the muscle is to be self-conscious and note the seemingly mundane things in the body. There are changes inside of the body, there could be a fat movement, a slight pain, a boil or acne, cold toes, stiffness or even shingles.

When changes are noted in the body and checked immediately, it prevents stress related illnesses. Gaining muscle is a lot to ask of yourself and yet the body does need to be lean to be fit. Gaining muscle cannot be taken lightly and should be taken seriously by adhering to regular health check-ups.

On how to gain muscle is to prevent side effects that may be linked to work outs and fat loss. The eyes may be deemed, the eyes may fluctuate and should be checked regularly. Natural or organic eye drops may cleanse out unwanted bacteria. The ears should also be cleansed as often as possible.

The cleansing are important because dirt increases as work increases. To keep a healthy body is a job in itself. Cleansing is a main factor when gaining the muscle and a key component in prolonging the life span.

Interestingly, Spirulina should be taken with Calcium and Magnesium despite its strength.

Dental appearance without pain and discomfort is one of the most delicate study on the planet. This is because of its greater need to discover a solution to the pain and tooth removal, after pain. Dental Occlusion is a discomfort that aggravates a need to remove the painful tooth or fill the tooth with metal such as mercury. But there are herbal mixes and combination that relieve pain of the tooth.

The question then is, should the tooth be removed every time it is in pain? How many teeth will be left? How can the pain be relieved in a longer time rather than fill the tooth with mercury that may lead to toxic problems in the stomach and digestive tract? Can the intestines survive much longer on swallowing metals?

There is a loss and blockage of the blood vessel when a tooth is damaged. The tooth cannot function properly, and it may not be receiving the proper circulation to keep it healthy. When the tooth is damaged, it is in pain, and it causes the gum to be in severe pain which may affect the rest of the teeth.

But how can the tooth be saved? The teeth can be in more pain after the gruesome removal of just one tooth. The removal of the tooth can result in more discomfort later on, in life.

Ensuring that the damaged tooth is repaired rather than removed, may increase the strength of the teeth dentition and the gum. This also improves the health of the throat, the esophagus, and its muscular tube.

When the teeth is in kept in good health with herbs, vitamins and minerals, infection is reduced; sore throat vanishes and rarely occurs, after a while. But which herbs are the best?

Which herbs have the right combination? The research is in depth but the cure is logical. The cure includes the brushing of the teeth with herbal toothpastes and organic mouth wash.

The natural flossing of the teeth is done by taking the right herbs such as Turmeric and Spirulina.

There is no one herb that can heal a tooth pain. This is achieved with the appropriate combination and the dose must be within the pain limit. When there is a severity in tooth pain, the immune system is not normal and therefore cannot receive a normal dose.

It will need a higher dose, to balance the pain and also regulate the immune system, which stops the pain.

A tooth pain causes ear pain and headache and this is where the study of Ashwagandha and the teeth steps in, gallantly.

This new study and discovery maintains the health of the teeth rather than the constant removal of it. As a result, the teeth is in constant connection with the brain and the brain cells without the stress and the instability of it.

CHAPTER EIGHTY-SIX

HEALTH STUDIES PAGE 1

Running Head: HEALTH ACROSS THE LIFESPAN
HEA 285 - HEALTH ACROSS THE LIFESPAN
WELLNESS PROJECT GUIDELINES
YOUR NAME:
INSTRUCTOR'S NAME:
CLASS INFORMATION:
DATE:

PART A

HEA 285 - Health Across the Lifespan
Wellness Project Guidelines
OBJECTIVE: Lifestyle that promotes
wellness on a longer term.
A lifestyle of Natural Health.
Regular check-ups, Herbal daily intake and yoga
Wellness is a time period when the body is energetic and ready to walk on, move on and work at a steady and acceptable pace.

To be in a state of wellness is to be fit to work and make a good living that is substantial and valuable to yourself as a person.

To be in a wellness state of mind, is to be alert and vigilant. The state of being in wellness is therefore related to a world where social activities are accepted as part of a healthy lifestyle.

The wellness state of mind is being able to understand the basics in politics, the basics of politics, being able to be registered to vote and being conscious of the social surroundings at any time and every time.

The state of wellness of mind is related to the economical lifestyle. A person is in that state of mind to balance the account, be conscious of their limitations and budget and be ready to make a list of priorities when buying and socializing.

The wellness of the mind is related to being at peace, thus avoiding unnecessary debts and crisis that may include carelessness.

The state of wellness of mind, creates in a person, the importance of being financially aware of their means at any time and live in that system in a comfortable way.

The state of wellness of mind is to be physically fit, physically clean and ready to work and be progressive in work and living standards.

PART B

Therefore, there is a sound basis to believe that the relativity between the social world, economical world, political world and financial world are interwoven and essential to a successful lifestyle on a longer term.

This particular aspect of my life where I like to be as energetic as possible, is of keen interest to me because I like to do a lot of research.

I like to be working all the time, creating ideas and making ideas into reality. Energy is critical to me, because without having the energy that is sufficient to produce lucrative output, there becomes a diminished lifestyle.

Energy gives me the power to study, research, move about and get things as I want them to. Therefore, a healthy lifestyle that includes yoga and herbal intake on a daily basis are one of life's most precious gifts.

Having daily vegetables, salads, protein drinks and well nourished dishes help me to be active and gain the strength that are vital and needed.

To avoid diabetes and other terminal illnesses, I take Spirulina.

According to Author P F Louis of the Natural Health News & Scientific Discovery, Spirulina gives strength and works as functional food to prevent diabetes.

(Study Touts Spirulina as Functional Food for Diabetes Management; www.naturalnews.com by P F Louis). Spirulina contains a lot of vitamins and minerals and is rich in Calcium.

Spirulina is fifty times stronger than Calcium and high in Vitamin B. There are various signs and warnings that contribute to my health firmness. When working or typing or even travelling, I realised that my stress levels become higher and become prone to high blood sugar, so I have spent many months and many years in creating a stable daily nutrition.

PART C

To avoid unnecessary health hazards, I have become more conscious of how far my body will take me at any given time. I have now cultivated a habit of regular herbal intake, regular exercise and the regular intake of sports nutrition. To be active is to be ready and steady and this improves my mentality and social outlook. I am able to make the right decisions especially on new projects.

Working too hard, without the balance of good food and nutrition creates problems when not needed.

This motto, I make for myself will then be: TO BE ACTIVE IS TO BE READY AND STEADY.

This has proven to be a supportive influence in my daily thoughts and has proven to be a positive push for my benefit. According to the Harvard Health Publications of the Harvard Medical School, it explains the importance and the basics of strength and power training and lists some good exercises that may help improve the body and the shape of the body.

(Strength and Power Training: A guide for adults of all ages by Harvard Health Publications;

www.health.harvard.edu).

Plan of Action as to maintaining my healthy lifestyle is to have a written daily plan whereby I have the activities I want, for each day. The possibility of adding a time or an estimated time period for every daily activity will be considered.

The daily necessity to exercise the neckline to ensure that the Thyroid glands are working properly cannot be underestimated.

The body's metabolism has to be working, at a good pace to ensure that the cholesterol is not too high and not too low. This is done by regular activities and the intake of protein essentials.

Preparing for new work, study and dimension also contributes to a steadier, better lifestyle.

PART D

According to the Medicine Net found on www.medicinenet.com, it explains why high cholesterol is dangerous to the health. When the heart muscles is not supplied with enough oxygen, it causes Atherosclerotic heart disease or narrowed coronary arteries.

The liver produces Cholesterol, however there is the bad cholesterol that blocks the arteries and then the blood vessels. Regular health check-ups and exercises such as yoga, skipping and bike riding may help reduce the bad fat in the body.

The blood supply to the brain must be adequate, it goes on to explain. In fact, the author explains that the larger carotid arteries must not be blocked in the neck to allow proper flow of blood to the brain. (Medical Author: Benjamin Wedro, MD, FACEP, FAAEM; Medical Editor: Charles Patrick Davies, MD, PHD; Title: Cholesterol Management,

Sub-title: Why is high Cholesterol dangerous? Website: MedicineNet.com)

In my six week journal, I have a goal that I have met. My goal for fitness and lifestyle varies annually. This time, the goal was to meet a two to three stone target, on my weighing scale.

To meet this target, I have done some gymnasium training and have had a regular yoga output. The first week showed the body adapting to my new fitness regime.

I became more energetic and could perform more chores as the weeks went by. My goal is to have a more stable sleep pattern and food nutrition but be prepared to adjust when in new places that I travel to.

My goal includes the watching of my cholesterol and ensuring that my lifestyle is balanced. I do some research on various herbal products that help with my cholesterol so that I can live a healthier life.

When my cholesterol is normal, I can breathe better, speak better and get more work done in good time.

Works Cited

Benjamin Wedro, MD, FACEP, FAAEM
Charles Patrick Davies, MD, PHD Cholesterol Management,
"Why is high Cholesterol dangerous?" <MedicineNet.com>
Cited on March 27, 2014. March 28, 2014
Harvard Health Publications

Strength and Power Training:
"A guide for adults of all ages by Harvard Health Publications"
<www.health.harvard.edu)>
Cited on March 27, 2014. March 28, 2014
LOUIS, P F

Natural Health News & Scientific Discovery
"Study Touts Spirulina as Functional Food for Diabetes
Management"
<www.naturalnews.com>
Cited on March 27, 2014. March 28, 2014.

SIX WEEKS JOURNAL: THE TRACKING OF DAILY FOOD,
EXERCISE, STRESS AND SLEEP MANAGEMENT

A SIX WEEK TRACKING FOR A HEALTHY, ENERGETIC LIFESTYLE is enormous but sets a daily goal that maintains a healthy lifestyle.	Eat three times a day. Have some snacks like low fat vegetable spring rolls. Some organic dairy products with the cereals. Hot chocolate drink after 6 pm daily.	Weeks 1 to 6 for 42 days is for a healthier lifestyle, to lower and balance my cholesterol levels. More energy is the target, increasing the metabolism in the thyroid glands is a target. Energy Health Strength Organics One Cigarette a day

TYPES OF FOOD: Organic foods and vegetables includes Broccoli, Cauliflower, Lettuce, Spinach, Country Mixed vegetables with some Organic Cottage pie, Brown rice, Brown bread, Organic butter spread, Organic goat milk and cheese. Side snacks and dessert will include some organic pudding, organic carrot cake, organic banana cake and some Olives. Rich organic oils and organic sauces with some rice and pasta.

BREAKFAST: Cereals, Organic Milk with Xylitol Sugar and some herbal vitamins such as Natural Vitamin C and Natural Vitamin B Complex.

LUNCH: Brown rice, Organic stew and fresh vegetables with protein drink and some herbal minerals such as Spirulina and Cod liver oil .

DINNER: Potatoes, Cabbage with Organic stew and protein drink and some herbal minerals and vitamins such as Evening Primrose Oil and Valerian root.

YOGA: Every thirty minutes a day. Preferably between 10 am and 11 am in the mornings.

NOTE: The herbs, vitamins and minerals prevent high blood pressure, high cholesterol and high blood sugar. Daily Drinks such as the energy drinks, Aloe Vera drinks and the Cranberry drinks are essential.

Stress	Yoga	The Bow which is a back bend	The Cat stretch which is to stretch the spine.	Take a herb for stress such as Valerian root that relaxes the muscles

Sleep	Some yoga	Some natural hot chocolate drink after 6 pm daily	Change bed including the mattress annually	Enjoy a ventilated room

Pulse rate jumped from 90 to 80	Heart rate improved and walking up and down the stairs did not get me out of breathe that quickly	Doing yoga exercises daily help improved the circulation of the legs, the mind is at peace	Eating a balanced diet, three times a day has given me a better direction. A good nutrition keeps me filled and strong	Getting the sleep that I needed was also significant and improved my skin appearance especially my face appearance	I realised that doing more of yoga rather than excess use of the gym gave me peace and steadiness

Analytic Findings	Regular yoga helps in the breakdown of fat	Exfoliating the skin improved the skin's complexion	Using organic Vitamin E creams brightened the skin and reduced the stress	The daily herbs improved and balanced my body's cholesterol levels.

Conclusion: A healthier lifestyle has been achieved. I reached my goal because I was able to stabilize my cholesterol levels. The results have been worth the effort because I am able to increase my energy and enjoy doing my tasks. I plan to continue this project, making new finds, trying new herbal products and trying some Karate, additionally to my yoga. I feel I look more youthful and I am able to gain some more confidence. It is a value for money lifestyle.

CHAPTER EIGHTY-SEVEN

ABOUT ME

NONA-MICHAEL ANKHESENAMUN JACKSON HEALTH &
HERBAL PROPOSAL

EXPERTISE

I am an Herbal Medicine, Dermatology and Dentistry Researcher.
Although I research vastly in herbs, I am also a Slogan writer, Lyricist,
Poet, Author, US Pro Se Attorney, Fashion Designer and Inventor.

I began to understand the herbal mixes when I became terminally
ill but went straight into remission within weeks.

The mixing of herbs has been a marvel over the years, however, I
discovered that herbs that heal and cure all terminal illnesses, do not
need to be mixed with inorganics to get the cure.

Ashwagandha is a most powerful herb in the world and can be
mixed with specific herbs, vitamins and minerals to achieve complete
recovery. This herb also heals skin cancer and problems and as a
matter of fact, works like a natural botox.

My Expertise on herbs is knowing and competently understanding
the herbs that combine well, to heal from a terminal illness. I have a
portfolio of herbs for documentaries on Social Media Instagram: @
sofia.richie8

It is widely believed that heart attack is the biggest killer, however,
we want to understand what really causes an attack or any terminal
illness. STRESS is the number one killer of all time. It is the awareness
of this illness called STRESS that will reduce many illnesses.

CAPABILITIES

I can mix herbs, vitamins and minerals to heal a terminal patient. I
can mix the herbs that will treat diabetes, which is becoming a harsh
illness that is becoming rampant. Diabetes makes a person feel they
have years to live but they are having years of torture.

I am able to treat skin cancer and skin cancer that may have been created from a diabetic complication. The treatment is highly likely to prevent an amputation.

I am able to advise on resuscitating a Cardiac Arrest patient using herbs, minerals and vitamins.

I am able to explain high doses for herbal mixes for any illness and for a surgery.

I am able to explain thoroughly, a test result for any illness and I am also able to indicate the herbal medicines needed and possibly how long the it may take for the recovery.

I am able to explain the elaborate processes of saving the teeth. Dentistry is more difficult so far and this is because the tooth can be in pain for many reasons. In fact, herbal mixes for the teeth, is my largest in my herbal catalogue. It is extensive and time consuming, but it is also worthy because the tooth is saved.

Removal of one tooth is not a guarantee that the rest of the teeth will not have some form of pain at some time. It is therefore better to save the tooth than remove it.

It is best to save the Pancreas than to have a transplant. It is best to prevent stress than have a terminal illness.

The combination to prevent illnesses is also elaborate because a person can prevent skin cancer but have a liver disease, perhaps because the herbs for the skin prevention is different from the liver prevention.

Amazingly enough, all the illnesses are linked and this is where I can combine the mixes in as accurate way as possible. But then, the dose is another concern. If the dose is not high enough or low enough, it may take a longer time to heal.

Toxicity is reduced when the herb for it, which is the same herb for resuscitating a heart patient, is added. Again, the dose always vary at all times.

My capability will also include gaining professional access to liquid herbs, in the case of an emergency.

I am able to lecture on the herbal subjects, carefully noting the highs and lows of exercises.

I would normally recommend yoga with the herbal intake.I am able to direct an obese person on the herbal method way, to slim down, without the loss of good fat. When good fat is shed during weight loss, it may lead to illnesses such as mental illness whereby the neurotransmitter is weakened and the Serotonin levels are so low, it causes great distress.

I am able to explain the importance of the Serum Globulin in blood and urine test results. A little over the expected result, can be a significant problem. I therefore can explain the link between the brain's Super Oxide and the Adrenal glands.

This is basically where the STRESS begins to build and yet the very place to prevent the major tragedy of a terminal illness.

I am able to explain the powerful importance of Vitamin B for all terminal illnesses and every day illnesses such as flu, cold, catarrh and sneezing. The link between sneezing and summer pollen count from flowers does not have to be a nightmare when the immune system is fed daily with the most appropriate herbs, vitamins and minerals.

TECHNOLOGY

I hope to propose my herbal mixes in bottles, powder, syrups, injections, IV drips, capsules, liquids, serum, drinks, foods, creams, lotions, energy drinks, slim fast drinks, milk shake drinks, documentary, frozen foods and ready meals.

I believe to understand that seed plantation is essential, as well as plant conservatory for in depth research into all herbs all over the world.

There is always a tree of life out there and Ashwagandha is only just one major herb that I have discovered amongst many others.

CHAPTER EIGHTY-EIGHT

NURSING HOME

Testosterone is a hormone in the body that regulates the normal function of the body. As older age begins, the testosterone is still needed. It is a hormone the body cannot do without.

To avoid nursing home and be Independent as an elderly person, there must be a balance. Can you afford to have anesthetics every three months or would it be better you stick to a regime with herbs that work as good as the testosterone pellets?

As older age is embraced, so are the questions that arise. A proper and written plan keeps the elderly in a place of balance. Learn to write out your plans in notebooks or in a diary.

Herbs, vitamins and minerals that are natural help maintain reasonable security. Make room for good hygiene. There is hygiene in the herbs. Whether for urinary incontinence or for osteoporosis, there is a cure.

Preparation for old age is vital. Can you avoid dependency on a walking stick? Using a walking stick is sometimes needed but if you take the herbs that build the bones, you can avoid osteoporosis and build a better spinal cord that sharpens the brain cells even at an older age.

Going to a nursing home should be temporary if you have to. Everyone has a problem and even nurses too have their own problems to resolve. But you can make life easier for yourself by taking control of your own problems. You know your own problems better than anybody else.

Herbs, vitamins and minerals are sold in herbal shops. So, learn to ask questions because they do provide Health advisors who can answer most of the questions.

There are also libraries with Library assistants who can look through books and the Internet to find out which herbs are good especially for walking because walking straight is one of the most critical problems in older age.

CHAPTER EIGHTY-NINE
OLD AGE

If you are able to continue the use of testosterone & pellets in old age, it is just as effective as the herbs. If you cannot cope with injections and quarterly anesthetic, then you should find the suggestions for herbs, vitamins and minerals useful at this time.

CHAPTER NINETY
OSTEOPOROSIS

Testosterone is a hormone that is produced by the body's testicles. Testosterone hormone contributes to the sex health and development of an individual.

Testosterone develops the bones and the muscle. However, a deficiency of testosterone may cause bones to soften, thin out and break. This causes Osteoporosis.

Taking synthetic and chemically induced medicines on a long scale may contribute to the weakening of the bones. The bones need to be cared for to regulate the testosterone levels in the body system.

The bones do not have to become weak because of old age rather, the bones can be kept stronger by taking herbs, vitamins and minerals.

CHAPTER NINETY-ONE

THE SPINAL CORD AND THE BONES

Herbs, vitamins and minerals such as Hydrolysed Collagen, Silica and Spirulina contribute to the density of the bones and the strength of the moving body.

The herbs, vitamins and minerals are there, to strengthen the spinal cord which weakens with age. This is what causes bending in some older people. The bones of the body need strength, the hips need to be fed with Iron supplements that are found in Spirulina.

CHAPTER NINETY-TWO
HERBS, VITAMINS AND MINERALS 1

Chromium Picolinate is a metal that increases the bone density. Caution should be taken when using the Chromium Picolinate because of its cancerous effect to the DNA. It should be combined with Brewer's Yeast and Vitamin B12.

Brewer's Yeast contains Chromium to aid weight loss and increase the bone density. It also increases lean muscle and keeps the body fit. But Brewer's Yeast must be taken with Vitamin B12 to increase the energy levels in the body.

Complete B complex is also good for Osteoporosis but should be combined with Brewer's Yeast because it does not contain Chromium. Complete B complex contains an active ingredient which is Folic acid responsible for the Spinal Cord strength. It prevents the Spinal Cord from dwindling and fracturing.

CHAPTER NINETY-THREE

ADRENAL FATIGUE 2

Testosterone is important in the life cycle of a person. Testosterone is needed for many important functions of the body. It gives strength, it strengthens the muscle, improves hair growth and encourages a healthy sex life.

Increased body fat from bad lipids can cause testosterone defects.

Testosterone pellet are derived from Soybeans so they are deemed as more of non-synthetic. As a result, testosterone pellets are deemed as reasonably safe when taken as injections although it may involve anesthetic procedure.

Americans call it Soybeans but the British call it Soyabeans.

Basically, Testosterone Pellet is more of botanical than herbal. That would mean that it includes plant parts that herbal may not, bark of trees, roots of the tree, seeds and the stem from the tree. The herbal and botanical are alike though, where nature and natural is concerned.

Testosterone pellet are said to be able to decrease bad fat and give brightness to the ailing skin.

Testosterone Pellet improves the sex drive, it also reduces depression and anxiety.

Testosterone Pellet has to be injected by a Health Expert however.

Testosterone Pellet works faster perhaps and because it is injected in the body system but then it has to be injected every three to four months.

If you don't like the idea of injections, there are other herbal ways of enjoying a good testosterone level. Perhaps you don't like the idea of having injections because you have to go through anesthetics.

There are herbs that contain Soybeans.

CHAPTER NINETY-FOUR

ADRENAL FATIGUE 2

Adrenal fatigue is when the top of the Kidneys are stressed out. The Adrenal glands carry out a lot of function in the body and endocrine system. As a result of their vast function to and from the brain, they can become a significant problem if they are in great stress or distress.

The powerful Indian herb called Ashwagandha can however regulate the adrenal glands.

CHAPTER NINETY-FIVE
CHRONIC FATIGUE 1

Testosterone pellet is made from soybean or soyabean. It has a botanical name called glycine max.

Soybean is used for restlessness and insomnia and that is what the testosterone pellet is for amongst many other functions.

Testosterone pellet and chronic fatigue would work hand in hand because of the soybean inside of it. It is possible that it lowers the cholesterol levels.

However the testosterone is injected in the body and re-injected after every three months. However there are other options such as swallowing herbs such as Ashwagandha, which is the equivalent of the Testosterone pellet.

The similarity between Testosterone pellet and Ashwagandha is that they both heal from cancer, restore the body's energy and activity. They both increase the testosterone levels and brighten the skin and the skin's colour.

Testosterone is always important in the body because it prevents osteoporosis as age ebbs in.

Testosterone pellet which is botanical in nature, is said to be used in Chinese Medicine to prevent colds and fevers.

Testosterone pellet functions like Phytosterols. Phytosterols work like cholesterol which means that they help stabilize the body's cholesterol levels. They would also regulate the muscle mass and increase the body's good fat.

Foods that contain Cholesterol are also called Phytosterols.

Testosterone pellet works as a phytoestrogen which makes it a moisturizer for the body especially the skin.

CHAPTER NINETY-SIX
CHRONIC FATIGUE

Chronic Fatigue is when a person is consistently exhausted for no apparent reason at all. The tiredness is not from work but is continuous.

Sometimes when a person over-works it could develop into Chronic Fatigue Syndrome.

To rectify this syndrome will be by reducing the bad fat in the body. The Testosterone pellet is for purposes that include the stabilizing of the cholesterol to reduce the chances of a heart attack or heart disease.

CHAPTER NINETY-SEVEN
FEMALE URINARY INCONTINENCE

What are Testosterone Pellets? Testosterone itself is a vital hormone that is needed in the body to be sexually productive, to gain muscle mass and to build the right energy.

Testosterone Pellets is said to boost testosterone in the body by injection. But then it is also said to have side effects.

So, how do you boost testosterone in the body without side effects? Are there ways to have Testosterone increased in the body without having to inject with Testosterone Pellets?

What is Female Urinary Incontinence? It is the loss of urine from the bladder at short notice. The urine comes out without being able to endure the extra minutes it should before getting into a bathroom. This may be that the urinary muscles have weakened from various reasons such as loss of vitamins, stress or from a terminal illness.

Testosterone can be increased in the body by taking the correct combination of herbs, vitamins and minerals. An overactive bladder that may have been caused by stress especially may be rectified especially when in the early stages.

Testosterone can be increased in various ways but must be done according to what the wishes are while keeping in mind, those facts that there are side effects in usage such as Testosterone Pellets.

The connection between Testosterone and Female Urinary Incontinence is that with stress comes a low libido and sex drive. The time is being spent on managing the urinary tract rather than enjoying the sex.

Taking Cranberry which is natural and a natural herb is an effective way of curing the leakages. Taking Cranberry with St John's Wort is one of the most powerful combinations ever.

St John's Wort relaxes the urinary tract muscle and Cranberry also controls the bladder leakage therefore, preventing the use of Catheter and similar.

CHAPTER NINETY-EIGHT
INFLAMMATION IN PSORIASIS AND ARTHRITIS

Testosterone pellet may decrease the inflammation in Psoriasis and Arthritis because it contains phytoestrogens.

Testosterone pellet is made of Soyoil so that it contains fatty acids that keep the skin and body supple. This would prevent Psoriasis and arthritis.

But what is Psoriasis? It is the inflammation of the skin which results in the scars, eczema, boils and sometimes loss of pigmentation. The inflammation of Psoriasis result in irritation and sometimes hallucinations.

Psoriasis is a detrimental problem to a person who has it. It could lead to pain and stiffness which is known as Psoriatic Arthritis.

CHAPTER NINETY-NINE
HERBS, VITAMINS AND MINERALS 2

There are herbs that keep the skin healthy such as Ashwagandha which should be taken with other herbs because of its high strength. It is a cancer healer on its own. Herbs such as Cod Liver Oil, Resveratrol, Garlic Oil, Pycnogenol, Complete B complex and Valerian Root.

There are various combination of herbs that make these healing successful. Vitamin C is known to heal the pain when combined with Ashwagandha. It reduces the arthritis and the redness as well as the itchiness of the skin. Ashwagandha also relieves from hallucinations and Paranoia Schizophrenia and mental illnesses that may result in this brutal itch caused by Psoriasis.

CAUSES OF PSORIASIS AND ARTHRITIS
Many factors may cause the psoriasis and arthritis. High blood sugar may have caused. Stress, being the number one killer of all time causes all diseases and illnesses.

Excess oil on the skin may result in tragic itching that develops into something more critical if not cared for immediately.

Dead skin cells accumulating in the bilirubin without detox may cause the inflammation. Whereas, the taking of Turmeric herb reduces the chances of toxins in the liver's bilirubin.

Excess cholesterol may be causing the itchiness. Taking the appropriate medication may help soothe this disease.

Avoid needles and injections if you can because Psoriasis and Arthritis sufferers have a longer healing process of the veins and the skin. Where possible use injections less frequently once you can.

CPSIA information can be obtained
at www.ICGtesting.com
Printed in the USA
BVOW08s0851211216

471499BV00001B/23/P

9 781681 228075